Management of Dementia:
Second Edition

Serge Gauthier
McGill Centre for Studies in Aging
Montreal, Québec, Canada

Clive Ballard
King's College London
London, UK

healthcare

New York   London

Informa Healthcare USA, Inc.
52 Vanderbilt Avenue
New York, NY 10017

© 2009 by Informa Healthcare USA, Inc.
Informa Healthcare is an Informa business

No claim to original U.S. Government works
Printed and bound in India by Replika Press Pvt. Ltd.
10 9 8 7 6 5 4 3 2 1

International Standard Book Number-10: 1-8418-4667-8 (Softcover)
International Standard Book Number-13: 978-1-8418-4667-5 (Softcover)
International Standard Book Number-13: 978-1-8418-4672-9 (Softcover) special edition

---

Library of Congress Cataloging-in-Publication Data

Gauthier, Serge, 1950–
    Management of dementia / Serge Gauthier, Clive Ballard. – 2nd ed.
        p. ; cm.
    Rev. ed. of: Management of dementia / Simon Lovestone. 2001.
    Includes bibliographical references and index.
    ISBN 978-1-84184-667-5 (softcover : alk. paper)   1. Dementia–Treatment.
I. Ballard, Clive.   II. Lovestone, Simon. Management of dementia..   III. Title.
    [DNLM: 1. Alzheimer Disease–diagnosis.   2. Alzheimer Disease–therapy.
3. Dementia–diagnosis.   4. Dementia–therapy.   5. Risk Factors.
WT 155 G276m 2008]
    RC521.G38 2008
    616.8'3–dc22   2008042441

For Corporate Sales and Reprint Permissions call 212-520-2700 or write to: Sales Department, 52 Vanderbilt Avenue, 16th floor, New York, NY 10017.

**Visit the Informa Web site at
www.informa.com**

**and the Informa Healthcare Web site at
www.informahealthcare.com**

Preface

The first edition of *Management of Dementia* has proven to be very useful to clinicians caring for persons with Alzheimer's disease and related disorders. Since 2001, there has been steady progress in this field, and all chapters have been updated with a clinical perspective based on the best available evidence.

The diagnostic criteria of Parkinson's disease dementia have been added to chapter 1. Behavioural disturbances cause a lot of distress to patients and caregivers, and continue to be a major management problem for clinicians, with considerable uncertainty as to the best overall approaches; we offer our advice in chapter 2 for the most troublesome behaviours, depression, psychosis and agitation, and in chapter 3 for sleep disturbances. Chapter 4 gives an update on the many genetic findings in Alzheimer's disease, Frontotemporal dementia and dementia with Lewy bodies. Chapter 5 on biological markers is complementary to chapter 1 on diagnosis. Chapters 6 and 7 on symptomatic and disease-modifying treatments discuss available drugs and potential preventive or stabilizing treatments. Chapter 8 offers advice for managing the difficult later stages of dementia in long-term care. Chapter 9 has been updated to include new assessment scales. Chapter 10 is a perspective on the management of dementia in the near future using primary and secondary prevention and drug treatments selected for individual patients with specific causes of dementia, treatments possibly based on the individual's phenotypic and genetic features.

We think that the care of persons with dementia and their caregivers has improved greatly in the past two decades, and we hope that this book will help further. We are not far from offering evidence-based prevention advice for persons at risk.

Serge Gauthier
Clive Ballard

Contents

Diagnosis

1

Introduction

There has been a shift in the past few years to persons consulting their physician because they are concerned about their risk of developing Alzheimer's disease (AD) or have minimal complaints. This is in addition to persons being brought in by family or friends with the more traditional symptoms of cognitive decline interfering with daily life, thus with dementia at different stages of severity. The physician or other health professional caring for persons with cognitive complaints must therefore be ready for quite a range of issues pertaining to diagnosis and treatment. This chapter will summarize the current clinical approach to the diagnosis of dementia, with additional information about persons who have memory complaints but no dementia.

Doctor, I am worried about getting Alzheimer like my mother did'

More and more persons in their midlife are consulting their physicians because they are concerned about their risk of AD later in their life. If they have any symptoms, they are minimal, such as losing tract of what they were looking for, delay in remembering someone's name. These persons perform well on screening tests such as the Mini Mental State Examination (MMSE; Folstein et al, 1975) supplemented by the Montreal Cognitive Assessment (MoCA; Nasreddine et al, 2005). Many will ask if there is 'a blood test' that can detect AD; there is currently no such test except for the rare families with early-onset, dominantly inherited AD (see chapter 4, 'Genetics'), although there is great interest in a blood marker for sporadic AD with adequate sensitivity and specificity (see chapter 5, 'Biomarkers').

These 'worried well' can be reassured that they do not have AD at this time, although they can have it later. We can estimate their risk relative to other individuals using variables derived from a population study and adding up into a 'midlife risk score' (Kivipelto et al, 2006), which identifies some excellent treatment targets for prevention (Panel 1.1).

Panel 1.1

Treatment targets for the prevention of dementia among middle-aged people*

- systolic BP < 140 mm Hg
- body-mass index < 30 kg/m^2
- total cholesterol < 6.5 mmol/L
- physical activity

*Modified from Kivipelto et al, 2006.

The advantage of looking systematically at such risk factors is that some can be modified by changes in lifestyle and interested persons can keep up to date with prevention strategies that include a Mediterranean diet (Scarmeas et al, 2006), building a social network (Bennett et al, 2006), leisure activities (Verghese et al, 2006), physical exercises (Larson et al, 2006), cognitive training (Willis et al, 2006) and one drink per day of alcohol or wine (Solfritti et al, 2007). Avoidance of certain risk factors in a prospective study in Japanese American middle-aged men was associated with a longer and healthier life (Willcox et al, 2006). It remains to be established if the prevalence of cognitive decline with age and dementia can be reduced using such population-based prevention strategy, which would be the most cost-effective way to reduce the burden of AD from a societal perspective (Brookmeyer et al, 2007). An illustration of a practical approach to prevention using a case study has been published by a workgroup of the Third Canadian Consensus Conference on the Diagnosis and Treatment Dementia (3CCCDTD; Patterson et al, 2008).

'Doctor, I am losing my memory'

Persons volunteering memory complaints and presenting themselves alone to their physicians rarely have dementia, but they are at risk of progressing towards one of the dementias

Panel 1.2
*Operational definition of mild cognitive impairment**

- *subjective memory complaints*
- *abnormal memory tests for age and level of education*
- *normal general cognitive performance*
- *normal activities of daily living*
- *not demented clinically*

*Petersen et al, 1999.

(predominantly AD). The large group of persons with 'mild cognitive impairment' (MCI) has attracted a lot of interest in the past decade since an operational definition was proposed by Petersen et al in 1999 (Panel 1.2). The latest expert conference on this topic was held under the auspices of the International Psychogeriatric Association (Gauthier et al, 2006), and the primary care physician perspective was studied by workgroups of the 3CCCDTD (Chertkow et al, 2007; Massoud et al, 2007) followed by a representative case study (Chertkow et al, 2008).

The clinical workup of someone with MCI is similar to any person with a cognitive complaint. It is preferable to get additional information from an informant (spouse, child, friend, co-worker) since informant-reported memory problems correlate better with cognitive outcomes (Carr et al, 2000). In other words, although most persons with MCI come alone to the physician's office, an informant should be found in order to get the best information possible on function at home or at work. The MMSE and the MoCA are done routinely by physicians or other health professionals. In-depth neuropsychological testing may be required in some individuals with high social or familial responsibility, where earlier recognition of executive impairment may require delegation of such responsibility.

There is currently no specific treatment for MCI. Cholinesterase inhibitors have been studied against placebo in thousands of persons with MCI, with no demonstrable benefit overall. The advice for prevention, mentioned in the previous section, is highly relevant for persons with MCI. Many will be interested in research programs aiming at secondary prevention.

'Doctor, does my wife have dementia?'

Most patients with dementia, even in mild stage, are brought in the physician's office by a family member. A careful history is the key to the clinical diagnosis of dementia, bringing out the components of the 'dementia of the AD type' defined in 1994 by the American Psychiatric Association (Panel 1.3).

The history is supplemented by a physical examination searching for evidence of peripheral vascular disease (hypertension, irregular pulse, carotid bruits) and of systemic conditions that could interfere with cognition and/or functional autonomy (goitre associated

Panel 1.3
Diagnostic criteria for dementia of the
Alzheimer's type*

Multiple cognitive deficits
- *in memory*
- *one or more of language, praxis, gnosis, executive functioning*

Causing
- *significant impairment and decline in social or occupational functioning*
- *gradual onset and continuing cognitive decline*

Not due to
- *other central nervous system or substance-induced conditions*
- *deficits not exclusively during course of delirium and not better accounted for by depression or schizophrenia*

Modified from American Psychiatric Association, 1994.

with hypothyroidism, for example), and a neurological examination looking for asymmetry in motor strength, tone and reflexes, which would suggest a focal lesion (stroke or tumour). Ancillary tests vary among countries, Canada likely being the least invasive in terms of laboratory investigations (Feldman et al, 2008).

'Doctor, does she have Alzheimer or dementia?'

Once the clinical diagnosis of dementia has been made, a differential diagnosis takes place,

using the best available information. The specific cause of dementia can often be positively identified from the pattern of symptoms as illustrated in Figure 1.1 for the typical patient with AD; the initial and transient change in mood is followed by a linear decline in cognitive and functional abilities, and then disruptive neuropsychiatric symptoms emerge followed by progressive rigidity, akinesia and gait instability.

The level of certainty for AD as a cause of dementia has been operationally defined by the National Institute of Neurological and Communicative Disorders and Stroke – Alzheimer's Disease and Related Disorders Association (NINCDS-ADRDA) in 1984: 'definite AD' requiring a brain biopsy or autopsy, 'probable AD' is similar to the APA criteria listed in Panel 1.3 and 'possible AD' indicates variations in the onset or course compared with typical AD, presence of a second brain disorder or systemic illness that is sufficient to cause dementia but that is not considered to be the cause of the dementia or a single gradually progressive deficit in the absence of other identifiable cause. (McKhann et al, 1984).

Each of the non-AD dementia has its own set of diagnostic criteria (Panels 1.4–1.7). Of particular clinical significance are the delirium-like fluctuating confusion and visual hallucinations in dementia with Lewy bodies (DLB) and dementia associated with Parkinson's disease (PDD), the early loss of

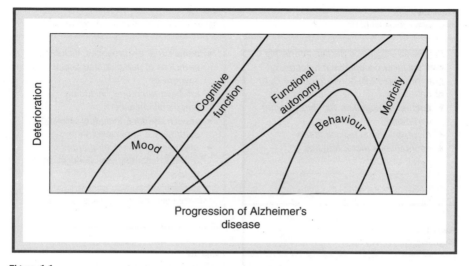

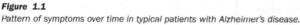

Figure 1.1
Pattern of symptoms over time in typical patients with Alzheimer's disease.

personal and social awareness combined with reduction in speech associated with fronto-temporal dementia and the stepwise deterioration with asymmetric neurological signs in vascular dementia.

The reality is that there is a lot of overlap between the different types of dementia: the majority of older patients with dementia have pathological features of AD, vascular disease and DLB/PDD (Schneider et al, 2007), with a marked overlap of Alzheimer and vascular changes almost inevitable over the age of 80 years (Lewis et al, 2006). This is important, as a lower burden of Alzheimer pathology is necessary to cause clinical dementia in the elderly in the presence of cerebrovascular

disease (Snowdon et al, 1997) and the concurrent vascular changes add to the cognitive impairment (Esiri et al, 1999).

The diagnosis of AD may be possible before the stage of dementia. A proposal has been made to update the NINCDS-ADRDA criteria and allow for an earlier diagnosis, combining clinical evidence of a progressive decline in episodic memory and laboratory evidence of abnormalities compatible with AD, using neuroimaging, spinal fluid examination, genetic testing (Dubois et al, 2007). Although currently meant only for research, it is likely that these criteria will make possible the diagnosis of AD one or two years earlier than traditionally possible.

Panel 1.4
Diagnostic criteria for DLB*

> Progressive cognitive decline interfering
> with social or occupational functioning
> one (possible DLB) or two (probable DLB)
> of
> • fluctuating cognition with pronounced
>   variations
> • recurrent visual hallucinations
> • spontaneous motor features of
>   parkinsonism
>
> ---
>
> *Modified from McKeith et al, 2005.

Panel 1.5
Diagnostic criteria for PDD*

> A dementia syndrome developing within
> the context of established Parkinson's
> disease, with
> • impairment in more than one cognitive
>   domain
> • decline from premorbid level
> • deficits severe enough to impair daily
>   life, independently of the impairment
>   ascribable to motor or autonomic
>   symptoms
>
> ---
>
> *Modified from Emre et al, 2007.

Panel 1.6
Diagnostic criteria for fronto-temporal dementia*

> • behavioural disturbances, including
>   early loss of personal and social
>   awareness
> • affective symptoms, including
>   emotional unconcern
> • speech disorder, including reduction,
>   stereotypy and perseveration
> • physical signs, including primitive
>   reflexes, incontinence, akinesia and
>   rigidity
>
> ---
>
> *Modified from Lund Manchester Groups,
> 1994.

Panel 1.7
Diagnostic criteria for vascular dementia*

> • decline in intellectual function
>   sufficient to interfere with activities of
>   daily life and not due to the physical
>   effects of stroke(s) alone
> • evidence by history, physical and/or
>   neuroimaging examination of stroke(s)
> • temporal relationship between
>   dementia and cerebrovascular disease
>
> ---
>
> *Modified from Chui et al, 1993, and Roman
> et al, 1994.

Should the diagnosis of dementia be made early?

Clearly yes, to clarify uncertainty about the nature of symptoms ranging from apathy and social withdrawal to mistakes in handling tasks at home or at work. Concomitant disorders such as depression and hypothyroidism, as well as vascular risk factors such as systolic hypertension, hypercholesterolemia and diabetes mellitus, can also be treated. Early diagnosis gives better opportunity to plan for the future. Symptomatic drugs can be offered and hopefully soon disease-modifying treatments will be available.

A more difficult question is the very early (pre-dementia) diagnosis of AD, if possible through the revised NINCDS-ADRDA criteria (Dubois et al, 2007); there is a risk of catastrophic reaction in someone with full understanding of the impact of diagnosis. Possibly, an approach similar to the one used in genetic screening clinics can be used, e.g., pre-testing assessment of how the earlier diagnosis would help or hinder the subject (Chao et al, 2008).

Should we tell patients what is the cause of their symptoms?

Yes. Most people dislike the term 'dementia' because it has the connotation of mental illness, thus patients and carers will prefer a 'disease' label. Using a good news/bad news approach, people are often reassured by the knowledge that there is a medical cause for the symptoms, and that specific drugs can be tried to relieve them. The lack of known genetic risk for children of patients with DLB may offer some relief, but this is not the case for AD (see chapter 4). The relatively stable course of vascular dementia compared to AD (at least in the short term) may also offer some additional hope.

Is there a right time to give the diagnosis?

As clinicians, we may suspect that a patient is progressing towards a dementia such as AD long before the symptoms reach diagnostic threshold. For instance, a long, postoperative, delirium could antedate AD by a number of years. A decline on serial MMSE scores could precede symptoms (Small et al, 2000). The converse is also true where families detect changes in mood, personality and initiative that they have seen associated with dementia in older relatives. If in doubt about the presence of dementia, it is better to state that it is not present at this time, but that follow-up is required once a year with attention to risk factors such as systolic hypertension. This may be a good time to 'put the papers in order' such as will and advance directives, when people are fully competent to do so, and identify who is likely to be the most significant family member to act as a carer, should the need arise. Once the diagnosis of dementia is clear in the clinician's mind and documented in his chart, this carer should be notified without delay. If the patient is in an angry denial stage, it may be better to give him or her disclosure in a stepwise approach (Fisk et al, 2007). Once insight into the significance of dementia has been lost in intermediate to late stages, there should be no hesitation about keeping the patient informed in clear but truthful language.

Should we tell patients with mild cognitive impairment that they may progress to dementia?

Yes, with the reassuring news that most persons with mild cognitive impairment as currently defined (Panel 1.2) do not progress to AD. Since up to 15% per year do progress to AD, interested patients can be referred to research sites running one of the many studies in this population.

Assessment of care needs

As a component of history taking towards the diagnosis of dementia, the clinician will have acquired knowledge of the functional abilities of the individual and of the resources available to cope with difficulties. For instance, someone may already be helping with finances and transportation. As part of a management strategy, additional information should be obtained on the person's life story, including work and leisure activities, as well as the quality of their social network, including family and close friends. Special attention will have to be paid to the carer, especially if older and frail, but also to a daughter or son caught between their responsibilities towards an elderly parent and their own children and spouse (the 'sandwich' effect). Family therapy or individual treatment for the distressed carer may be needed. Referral to a local Alzheimer society, whatever the cause of dementia, is an important step in the education of patients and carers (Brodaty and Berman, 2007). Referral to local community-based formal support services for help at home and access to support groups, day programs and respite care

is another useful step, often underused by families (Katofsky, 2007).

Prognosis

The natural history of AD can be understood as a series of milestones that can be used in clinical trials as outcome, or in patients' and caregivers' education (Galasko et al, 1995; Panel 1.8).

There have been many attempts to predict which patients will do better or worse (Sarazin et al, 2007). A list derived from many publications for clinical features that predict a rapid decline is shown in Panel 1.9.

The clinician will have to schedule closer visits on follow-up of patients in the rapid-decline category, give advance warning of things to come, and facilitate planning for the carer, all the way to nursing-home placement. An example of how such cases may

Panel 1.8
Milestones in progression of dementia*

- *conversion from mild cognitive impairment to dementia*
- *loss of instrumental activities of daily living (ADL)*
- *emergence of neuropsychiatric symptoms*
- *nursing home placement*
- *loss of self-care ADLs*
- *death*

*Modified from Galasko et al, 1995.

Panel 1.9
Clinical features suggestive of rapid decline

- aphasia, severe
- caregiver psychological morbidity
- concomitant vascular disease
- extra-pyramidal signs, early
- greater age
- myoclonus, early
- non-AD dementias
- psychosis, early
- unmarried men

Panel 1.10
Reasons to consider referral to a specialist*

- continuing uncertainty about the diagnosis after initial assessment and follow-up
- request by family or patient for second opinion
- presence of significant not responsiveness to treatment
- intolerance or lack of response to disease-specific pharmacotherapy
- need for additional help for patient management or caregiver support
- need to involve other health professionals, voluntary agencies, or local service providers
- when genetic counselling is indicated
- when research studies into diagnosis or treatment are being performed

*Patterson et al, 1999.

pan out follows. A woman practicing family medicine in her mid-fifties is brought to her physician by her husband because of mistakes at work over the past year. She has significant difficulties expressing herself in her second language and is reverting to her mother tongue, not well understood by the spouse. Myoclonus is visible in her limbs. The diagnosis of AD is made, confirmed by consultation with a specialist, and the spouse is warned of the poor prognosis. There was no improvement on a cholinesterase inhibitor, and she needed nursing-home placement 1 year later. The spouse had taken a year off work to care for her at home, and was able to go back to teaching. She died a year later from pneumonia.

Referral to specialist services

Although family practitioners have a central role in the diagnosis and management of dementia, they will face uncertainty in some patients with very early symptoms, atypical presentations of AD, or rare types of dementia. Some of the management issues need a team approach, both in the community and in institutions. Guidelines have been prepared to suggest when to refer to a specialist (Panel 1.10).

Summary

- Family practitioners play a key role in the diagnosis and management of people with dementia and their carers.
- Practitioners have responsibility for disclosure of diagnosis, assessment of care needs, and prognosis.

- Carers and practitioners can and should call upon a number of resources in their community.

References

American Psychiatric Association (1994). *Diagnosis and statistical manual of mental disorders*, 4th edn. Washington DC: APA.

Bennett DA, Schneider JA, Tang Y, Arnold SE, Wilson RS (2006). The effect of social networks on the relation between Alzheimer's disease pathology and level of cognitive function in old people: a longitudinal cohort study. *Lancet Neurol* 5, 406–412.

Brodaty H, Berman K (2007). Caregiver support: support of families. In: Gauthier S, ed. *Clinical diagnosis and management of Alzheimer's disease*, 3rd edn. London, UK: Informa Healthcare, 279–298.

Brookmeyer R, Johnson E, Ziegler-Graham K, Arrighi HM (2007). Forecasting the global burden of Alzheimer's disease. *Alzheimers Dement* 3, 186–191.

Carr DB, Gray S, Baty J, Morris JC (2000). The value of informant versus individual's complaints of memory impairment in early dementia. *Neurology* 55, 1724–1726.

Chao S, Roberts JS, Marteau TM, Silliman R, Cupples LA, Green RC (2008). Health behavior changes after genetic risk assessment for Alzheimer disease: the REVEAL study. *Alzheimer Dis Assoc Disord* 22, 94–97.

Chertkow H, Massoud F, Nasreddine Z, et al (2008). Diagnosis and treatment of dementia: 3. Mild cognitive impairment and cognitive impairment without dementia. *CMAJ* 178, 1273–1285.

Chertkow H, Nasreddine Z, Joanette Y et al (2007). Mild cognitive impairment and cognitive impairment, no dementia: part A, concept and diagnosis. *Alzheimers Dement* 3, 266–282.

Chui HC, Victoroff JI, Margolin D, et al (1993). Criteria for the diagnosis of ischemic vascular dementia proposed by the State of California Alzheimer's Disease Diagnostic and Treatment Centres. *Neurology* 42, 473–480.

Dubois B, Feldman HH, Jacova C, et al (2007). Research criteria for the diagnosis of Alzheimer's disease: revising the NINCDS-ADRDA criteria. *Lancet Neurol* 6, 734–746.

Emre M, Aarsland D, Brown R, et al (2007). Clinical diagnostic criteria for dementia associated with Parkinson's disease. *Mov Disord* 12, 1689–1707.

Esiri MM, Nagy Z, Smith MZ, Barnetson L, Smith AD (1999). Cerebrovascular disease and threshold for dementia in the early stages of Alzheimer's disease. *Lancet* 354, 919–920.

Feldman HH, Jacova C, Robillard A, et al (2008). Diagnosis and treatment of dementia: 2. Diagnosis. *CMAJ* 178, 825–836.

Fisk JD, Beattie BL, Donnelly M, Byszewski A, Molnar FJ (2007). Disclosure of the diagnosis of dementia. *Alzheimers Dement* 3, 404–410.

Folstein MF, Folstein SE, McHugh PR (1975). "Mini-Mental State": a practical method for grading the cognitive state of patients for the clinician. *J Psychiat Res* 12, 189–198.

Galasko D, Edland SD, Morris JC, Clark C, Mohs R, Koss E (1995). The Consortium to Establish a Registry for Alzheimer's Disease (CERAD). Part XI. Clinical milestones in patients with Alzheimer's disease followed over 3 years. *Neurology* 45, 1451–1455.

Gauthier S, Reisberg B, Zaudig M, et al (2006). Mild cognitive impairment. *Lancet* 367, 1262–1270.

Katofsky L (2007). Community-based formal support services. In: Gauthier S, ed. *Clinical diagnosis and management of Alzheimer's disease*. 3rd edn. London, UK: Informa Healthcare, 299–314.

Kivipelto M, Ngandu T, Laatikainen T, Winblad B, Soininen H, Tuomilehto J (2006). Risk score for the prediction of dementia risk in 20 years among middle aged people: a longitudinal, population-based study. *Lancet Neurol* 5, 735–741.

Larson EB, Wang L, Bowen JD, et al (2006). Exercise is associated with reduced risk for incident dementia among persons 65 years of age and older. *Ann Intern Med* 144, 73–81.

Lewis H, Beher D, Cookson N, et al (2006). Quantification of Alzheimer pathology in ageing and dementia: age-related accumulation of amyloid-beta(42) peptide in vascular dementia. *NeuropatholAppl Neurobiol* 32, 103–118

Lund and Manchester Groups (1994). Clinical and neuropathological criteria for fronto-temporal dementia. *J Neurol Neurosurg Psychiatry* 57, 416–418.

McKhann G, Drachman D, Folstein M, et al (1984). Clinical diagnosis of Alzheimer's disease: report of the NINCDS-ADRDA Work Group under the auspices of Department of Health and Human Services Task Force on Alzheimer's Disease. *Neurology* 34, 939–944.

McKeith IG, Dickson DW, Lowe J, et al.; for the Consortium on DLB (2005). Dementia with Lewy Bodies: Diagnosis and Management. Third Report of the DLB Consortium. *Neurology* 65, 1863–1872.

Massoud F, Bellevile S, Bergman H, et al (2007). Mild cognitive impairment and cognitive impairment, no dementia: part B, therapy. *Alzheimers Dement* 3, 283–291.

Nasreddine ZS, Phillips NA, Bédirian V, et al (2005). The Montreal Cognitive Assessment, MoCA: a brief screening tool for Mild Cognitive Impairment. *J Am Geriatr Soc* 53, 695–699.

Patterson C, Feightner JW, Garcia A, et al (2008). Diagnosis and treatment of dementia. 1. Risk assessment and primary prevention of Alzheimer disease. *CMAJ* 178, 548–556.

Patterson C, Gauthier S, Bergman H, et al (1999). The recognition, assessment and management of dementing disorders: conclusions from the Canadian Consensus Conference on Dementia. *CMAJ* 160(suppl), S1–S20.

Petersen RC, Smith GE, Waring SC, Ivnik RJ, Tangalos EG, Kohmen E (1999). Mild cognitive impairment: clinical characterization and outcome. *Arch Neurol* 56, 303–308.

Roman GC, Tatemichi TK, Erkinjuntii T, et al (1994). Vascular dementia: diagnostic criteria for research studies: report of the NINCDS-AIREN international workshop. *Neurology* 43, 250–260.

Sarazin M, Horme N, Dubois B (2007). Natural decline and prognostic factors. In: Gauthier S, ed. *Clinical diagnosis and management of Alzheimer's disease*. 3rd edn. London, UK: Informa Healthcare, 137–148.

Scarmeas N, Stern Y, Tabg MX, Mayeux R, Luchsinger JA (2006). Mediterranean diet and risk for Alzheimer's disease. *Ann Neurol* 59, 912–921.

Schneider JA, Arvanitakis Z, Bang W, Bennett DA (2007). Mixed brain pathologies account for most dementia cases in community-dwelling older persons. *Neurology* 69, 2197–2204.

Snowdon DA, Greiner LH, Mortimer JA, Riley KP, Greiner PA, Markesbery WR (1997). Brain infarction and the clinical expression of Alzheimer disease. The Nun Study. *JAMA.* 277, 813–817.

Solfritti V, D'Introno A, Colacicco AM, et al (2007). Alcohol consumption, mild cognitive impairment, and progression to dementia. *Neurology* 68, 1790–1799.

Verghese J, LeValley A, Derby C, et al (2006). Leisure activities and the risk of amnestic mild cognitive impairment in the elderly. *Neurology* 66, 821–827.

Willcox BJ, He Q, Chen R, et al (2006). Midlife risk factors and healthy survival in men. *JAMA* 296, 2343–2350.

Willis SL, Tennstedt SL, Marsiske M, et al (2006). Long-term effects of cognitive training on everyday functional outcomes in older adults. *JAMA* 296, 2805–2814.

Behavioural disturbances

2

'Doctor, she wants to hit me when it's time for her bath'

The major neuropsychiatric syndromes occurring as part of AD include behavioural symptoms such as aggression, abnormal eating, apathy, agitation, disinhibition, restlessness, shouting and other behaviours likely to give rise to difficulties for the patient or others, as well as psychiatric disorders such as depression, anxiety and psychosis. Other psychiatric syndromes including mania, obsessive-compulsive disorders and even alcohol dependence are also found, but are much less frequent. Eliciting psychiatric symptoms and assessing behavioural disturbance can be difficult in people with dementia as it is largely dependant on the caregiver and may differ between family and professional carers (Lukovits and McDaniel, 1992) and reflects the interaction between the patient and the environment.

In this chapter, we concentrate on aggression, agitation, depression and psychosis, as the most frequent and troublesome neuropsychiatric and behavioural syndromes. Although we do suggest some treatment approaches, we note, as others have before us, the lack of data on which to establish evidence-based guidelines. It is disappointing that almost a century after Alzheimer and Auguste that this is the case.

Depression

Prevalence and cause of depression in dementia

Of all the psychiatric syndromes to occur in AD, depression is the most common. However, it has proven difficult to establish just how common depression is, almost certainly because of the obvious difficulty in deciding how to assess altered mood in an individual with cognitive deficits. This problem is not restricted to academic studies. Just as it can be difficult to measure depression in a research setting, so too in a clinical setting. Inevitably, some depression in patients with dementia will not be recognised and equally some patients will be treated for depression with little effect. There is a nosological problem too: many of the behavioural manifestations of depression – altered activity and energy level, decreased appetite and altered circadian rhythms – are also manifest in dementia syndromes without any suggestion of changed mood. Nonetheless, despite these difficulties, scales, such as the Cornell Scale for Depression in Dementia, have been successfully developed to rate depression in AD (Vida et al, 1994). Diagnosing depression can be particularly difficult in people with severe dementia, where the individuals have a limited capacity to describe their symptoms or feelings and the differential diagnosis from apathy and agitation with an effective component

can be very difficult at this stage of the disease.

Most studies find a high rate of depression in patients with AD. A third or more may have symptoms of depression (Aarsland et al, 1996; Starkstein et al, 1997; Starkstein et al, 1995; Lyketsos et al, 1997b; Migliorelli et al, 1995; Burns et al, 1990a) and a fifth may have a major depressive episode (Lyketsos et al, 1997a, 1997b; Burns et al, 1990a; Starkstein et al, 1997;). Rates may be lower in community samples (Lyketsos et al, 2000a, 2000b). Historically, it has always been held that depression is more common in vascular dementia and, indeed, there is some research evidence to substantiate this, suggesting a higher frequency (Reichman and Coyne, 1995, Lyketsos et al, 2000a, Ballard et al, 2000a). Other studies of mildly affected individuals (Verhey et al, 1995), however, do not show greater rates of depression in vascular versus AD dementias. It might be that depression in vascular dementia is different to that of AD – more persistent and less clearly related to level of cognitive decline than in AD (Fischer et al, 1990; Ballard et al, 1996). Research studies fairly consistently report higher frequencies in dementia with Lewy bodies (DLB) (e.g. Ballard et al, 1999, Klatka et al, 1996) and Parkinson's disease dementia (PDD) (Aarsland et al, 2001) than in AD.

The weight of evidence, research and clinical, is that depressive symptoms are common in AD, and probably even more frequent in vascular dementia, DLB and PDD. Importantly, there is less certainty about how frequently this amounts to a full and major depressive episode, and certainly a substantial proportion of mild depressive episodes may be transient (Ballard et al, 1996). From the practical perspective, depression results in major negative impact upon both patients and their carer and yet is potentially treatable. It seems appropriate to err on the side of over-diagnosis of depression in AD; the price of over-treatment is small compared with the potential consequences of not treating at all.

The relation between depression and AD is actually even more complex than suggested by the studies cited earlier. A large body of epidemiological research has suggested that depression may actually be a risk factor for AD – a history of depression being more common in those with AD (Devanand et al, 1996; Jost and Grossberg, 1996; Jorm et al, 1991; Kessing and Andersen, 2004; Speck et al, 1995). The timing of the depression to the onset of AD is critical; if the depression occurred only a few years before, then it could be that the altered mood was a prodromal feature of AD, and not a risk factor for dementia. Some other neurodegenerative conditions such as Huntington's disease have a wide range of psychiatric syndromes that can occur as a prodromal feature (Lovestone et al, 1996). The question whether AD has a depressive prodromal phase is also not resolved as yet. In a study of twins, it was shown, for example, that depression increased the risk of AD but that this risk increased the closer the timing of the depression and dementia, suggesting, in this study at least, that most of the apparent increase in risk was due to a prodromal syndrome (Steffens et al, 1997). However, other studies find a preservation of the risk effect even when the depression occurred more than a decade before the dementia (Speck et al, 1995) and it is difficult to envisage a prodrome lasting as long as this. There are many other potential overlaps including the rare but important condition of depressive pseudodementia (Fischer, 1996) and the potential impact of subcortical cerebrovascular disease as a substrate of both depression (Godin et al, 2008) and cognitive impairment (O'Brien, 2006).

Why is it that only some people with AD get depressed? The answer to this question may tell us something interesting about either dementia or depression, and so researchers have compared depressed AD patients with non-depressed AD patients according to a variety of measures. Perhaps the most interesting finding was that of Pearlson et al (1990), who found that patients with depression have more relatives affected by depression than did demented but not depressed patients. This suggests that a genetic factor may alter the chances of being depressed. The *APOE 4* gene that is associated with AD itself does not seem to be a genetic risk factor for depression in AD (Lyketsos et al,

1997a; Cacabelos et al, 1996, Lopez et al, 1997). Polymorphisms associated with alteration in 5-HT2 A and 5-HT2 receptors may be more important. In an important recent study, carriers of the 5-HT2 A C102 allele were five times more likely to have major depressive illness than heterozygotes in the context of AD, and homozygous or hemizygous carriers of the 5-HT2 C Ser allele were 12 times more likely to have major depressive illness than homozygous or hemizygous carriers of the 5-HT2 C Cys allele (e.g. Holmes et al. 1998, 2003). In addition to genetic factors, patterns of neuronal loss may be important. It is possible that people with AD developing depression have a particular loss of neurons that are known to alter mood, such as the adrenergic or serotenergic neurons (Forstl et al, 1992; Chen et al, 1996), although this has not been confirmed in more robust studies (Hoogendijk et al, 1999). Alternatively, clinical experience suggests that some people's personality type is accentuated after developing dementia and that premorbid personality may be a risk factor for becoming depressed after the dementia starts. Some evidence does support this idea but it is difficult to tell whether this is relatives reassessing personality after the patient becomes depressed or whether it is a true association (Strauss et al, 1997). It is commonly thought, and might be expected, that in the early stages some individuals experience lowered mood as a result of their understanding about the disease and their own future. However, our own clinical experience suggests that whilst an important consideration, this is less common than might be expected. We find that patients respond rather well to be told of the diagnosis and even prognosis and rarely become depressed as a direct result of being told.

Case study

Two elderly brothers had lived together since the death of the wife of the oldest brother; the other brother had never married. For many years they coexisted quite happily, they had been close for much of their lives and had always lived within a few hundred yards of each other. The youngest brother by three years was known to have had AD for more than 2 years and within the past 6 months it became increasingly apparent to the family doctor that the oldest of the two also had memory loss. A referral was made to specialist services. On assessment, it became apparent that both brothers had AD, of mild severity in the older and moderate severity in the younger. In addition, both appeared miserable and the carers (a sister who visited often and the children of the older brother) reported that both brothers spent much of the day slumped in chairs facing each other. The younger brother was unable to describe his mood but was losing weight, had no energy, and looked miserable. He often said that he wished he was dead. The older brother described feeling miserable and was seen crying frequently. Both brothers slept poorly. A management plan was instigated that included an improved home-care package and regular attendance at a day unit with structured activities. An antidepressant was commenced for both brothers. Six months later the older brother, while not cheerful, was no longer as miserable as before. The younger brother continued to look as miserable as previously but was active, sleeping well and putting on weight.

Assessment of depression in dementia

The case history above shows a few of the problems in diagnosing depression in a person with AD, not least because many of the symptoms of depression also occur in dementia. Inherent biases also make diagnosis difficult; physicians can be slow to recognise depression as part of a dementia syndrome and caregivers can ascribe symptoms of the dementia to depression. Nonetheless, as for behavioural disturbance, the assessment of depressive symptomatology starts with a careful history from the informant. The symptoms of depression in AD are the same as those in older people without dementia but the most important aspect of assessment is change – has there been a change in mood, has there been a change in activity? The onset of a new symptom suggestive of depression in someone with an established dementia is a very important observation to make. Some of the areas to consider in the assessment of depression in dementia are illustrated in Panel 2.1. Caregivers can be reliable informants of depression in AD (Victoroff et al, 1997), although repeated studies have

Panel 2.1
Assessment of depression in dementia

Mood
- *Do the patients say that they feel depressed or unhappy?*
- *Do they look depressed or cry frequently?*
- *Is there diurnal variation in mood (worse in the morning)?*
- *Does the patient still enjoy the things they used to enjoy (a sing-song; visit of grandchildren)?*

Speech
- *Has speech reduced in rate or volume?*
- *If the patients normally sing or hum, do they still do so?*

Activity
- *Has activity declined, does the patient seem to lack energy?*
- *Is the patient overactive; do they wring their hands or act similarly?*
- *Does activity change during the day; is the patient worse in the morning?*

Sleep
- *Has the pattern of sleep changed?*
- *Is there a regular disturbance of night-time sleeping; if so is it early morning waking?*

Appetite
- *Has appetite changed; is there weight loss?*

shown that caregivers report higher levels of depression than do trained observers. Scales can also be an addition to routine clinical practice; the Cornell Scale for Depression in Dementia (Alexopoulos et al, 1988) is a particularly useful observer-rated scale, although it is a measure of depression severity rather than a screening instrument. In clinical practice, however, a combined approach of careful assessment and observation of the patient, an interview with an informant concentrating upon change, together with judicious use of rating scales is the most effective means of detecting depression in AD.

The effects of depression in AD

Quality of life in dementia can be difficult to measure (see chapter 9), but all working in the field, both formal and informal carers, agree that good quality of life is not only desirable but is also achievable. There is no question that depression results in a poor quality of life and experiencing depression during the course of dementia is nothing short of a tragedy. However, apart from the consequences for the patient, it is increasingly clear that depression affects the patient's care needs and also has a major impact upon carers. Patients with depression will function at a level below their ability as a consequence of reduced energy and motivation and require increasing support. Assessments of activity (daily living skills) do

show that function is impaired in patients with depression (Lyketsos et al, 1997a, 1997b; Fitz and Teri, 1994) and there is some evidence that depression is one factor leading to aggression (Lyketsos et al, 1999; Victoroff et al, 1998). Carers find the associated symptoms of AD – the behavioural disturbance and psychiatric problems – far harder to cope with than the disease itself. Carers of people with AD are themselves significantly more likely to be depressed and anxious than carers of people without depression (Donaldson et al, 1998; Brodaty and Luscombe, 1998).

Treating depression in AD

Treating depression in AD is difficult, particularly when the symptoms tend to persist or recur (Levy et al, 1996; Starkstein et al, 1997). When recognised, however, depression should be treated energetically and in many cases, especially in those patients with milder depression, the symptoms can be alleviated or removed entirely. It is important to exclude any medical disorders or drug therapies which could be contributing to depression. Where no such factors are identified, a combination of both pharmacological and psychological therapeutic approaches is often the best approach for moderate or severe depression, but there is, unfortunately, little evidence from well-conducted studies on which to base a therapeutic programme. This is one of the most important omissions in AD research;

while clinical experience can guide us to effective treatments, it would be extremely useful to have randomised trial data on which to base guidelines for these most debilitating symptoms.

Limited but important evidence suggests that non-pharmacological approaches such as cognitive–behavioural therapy, pleasant activities and exercise may have significant benefits in the treatment of depression in people with AD (Teri et al, 1997; Teri et al, 2003). Other measures may also affect both the patients and their carer – interesting work is being done to examine the interactive style between carers and patients (Fearon et al, 1998; Vitaliano et al, 1993). Attendance at a day centre specialising in dementia care can also help. Non-pharmacological approaches can be very simple and should probably be the treatment of choice for mild-to-moderate transient depression.

Several tricyclic antidepressants have been examined in clinical trials for the treatment of depression in people with Alzheimer's disease, with limited evidence of benefit (Reifler et al, 1989; Petracca et al, 1996), perhaps in part because the anticholinergic side effects may have a more detrimental impact than any treatment benefits. More recent studies with selective serotonin reuptake inhibitors (SSRIs) such as sertraline and escitalopram have indicated better tolerability and generally a more favourable response to treatment (Gottfries et al, 1992; Burke et al, 1997; Katona et al, 1998; Lyketsos et al, 2000b; Lyketsos

et al, 2003; Cipriani et al, 2009), although the evidence from a formal meta-analysis highlights that the benefit of treatment of depression in dementia is still far from clear (Bains et al, 2008). Although serotonin and noradrenaline reuptake inhibitors (SNRIs) are often prescribed, there is no evidence to support their use in these patients.

It should also be noted that clinical trials often exclude more severely depressed patients, which probably reduces the apparent treatment benefit in these studies. It should also be emphasised that the limited evidence from clinical trials should not be used as a reason to withhold antidepressant treatment from a patient with AD who is severely depressed.

The choice of antidepressant drug is important because patients with dementia are often frail and may be expected to be more susceptible to side effects. Falls, possibly due to orthostatic hypotension (a fall in blood pressure on rising) and increased confusion in particular, are a problem with the tricyclic antidepressants. There is another reason to favour the newer SSRI compounds, however. AD is a cholinergic disorder in that the cholinergic neurons are lost first and most in the course of the disorder. The first available antidementia drugs are cholinergic agents. Tricyclic antidepressants have a major anticholinergic effect and would be expected to hasten decline. Neuroleptics also have similar anticholinergic effects and are associated with a more rapid deterioration in cognition (McShane et al, 1997; Holmes et al, 1997). For this reason, we would recommend that only drugs without significant anticholinergic activity be used to treat depression in dementia; in practice this means that treatments should only be considered with an SSRI or related antidepressant. Therapy should be started early, as soon as depression is suspected. Many, perhaps most, patients can be treated in the community but at times it can be helpful to admit a patient to an inpatient facility to ensure compliance and to instigate other therapies. Certainly admission to an inpatient unit as a short-term measure can be successful (Zubenko et al, 1992). The outcome of therapy should be monitored carefully; the report of the carer is probably the most effective means by which to judge the effectiveness of treatment.

Although successful in many cases, there is a placebo effect associated with antidepressant therapy, even in those with dementia. Given that the outcome is often assessed partly or in whole through the carer, then it may be that the placebo effect is with the carers themselves – they feel something is being done, this reduces their own levels of stress, and this either has an effect on the patient or affects the carer's view of the patient's mood. For people residing in care homes or nursing homes, attention to care plans to increase social interaction and pleasant activities may be extremely effective for milder depression. In the absence of any specific evidence relating to

the treatment of depression in vascular dementia or DLB, the same treatment approaches as recommended for AD are probably the best guide for clinical practice.

Mania

Elevated mood is very rare in AD, occurring in less than 4% of patients in the few studies to examine this (Burns et al, 1990a; Lyketsos et al, 1995). However, it does occur, and can present major management difficulties.

Case study

The husband of a 68-year-old retired occupational therapist (OT) complained to his family doctor that his wife was awake all night and was irritable and aggressive with him. The family doctor visited and then referred the patient to specialist services as a case of hypomania. The patient herself did indeed display many of the features of hypomania. She was very active and found it difficult to sit down. She was dressed in very bright clothes and, according to her husband, this was highly unusual for her. Her make-up was also exaggerated – vivid blue eyeshadow, thickly applied rouge and a dramatic red lipstick. All were new purchases. She described herself as feeling fantastic but on examination her mood was more irritable than elevated. There were no hallucinatory experiences but she did claim to be head OT of a nearby hospital, was writing a text book on the subject, and had plans to start an OT school in her flat. These changes in her appearance and character had all occurred within the previous month, but in discussion with her husband it became apparent that for at least the past 6 months she had been doing less around the house and her husband and his oldest daughter had gradually taken on most of the shopping, cooking and cleaning. Neither he nor his daughter had noticed any memory problems and in her current state it proved impossible to do cognitive testing. She was admitted and treated with a combination of lithium and neuroleptics and made a gradual recovery. However, as soon as she was admitted, it was apparent that she had difficulty in orientating herself and could never find the bathroom, leading to incontinence on several occasions. As her mood disturbance subsided, the extent of her cognitive impairment became clear – she scored 16/30 on Mini Mental State Examination. A discharge home with a comprehensive care package was only temporarily successful and within 4 months of discharge she needed to be placed in a nursing home.

Psychosis and agitation

Prevalence and causes of agitation and psychosis in dementia

Aggression and non-aggressive agitation occur in about 20% of people with Alzheimer's disease (AD) in contact with clinical services (Burns et al, 1990c) or living in the community (Lyketsos et al, 2000a, 2000b) and 40% to 60% of people in care facilities (Margallo-Lana et al, 2001). Common symptoms include verbal aggression, physical aggression, restlessness and shouting, often presenting in a very situation-specific way, such as physical or verbal aggression occurring during personal care. Psychosis, both hallucinations and delusions, are also common in AD patients, occurring in 10% to 50% of patients in contact with clinical services (Levy et al, 1996; Drevets and Rubin, 1989; Burns et al, 1990b) or in nursing homes (Margallo-Lana et al, 2001), but with a lower frequency in the community (Lyketsos et al, 2000a, 2000b). Psychotic phenomena do not have the same quality as those that occur in primary psychotic disorders such as schizophrenia. For example, delusions of theft are very common; whether a person with dementia believing someone has come into the house to steal belongings that have been misplaced is not really comparable to the person with schizophrenia having a complex paranoid delusion. First rank symptoms are extremely rare in people with Alzheimer's disease, as are the delusions of partition and elaborate paranoid ideation that are common in late onset schizophrenia (Ballard et al, 1995). Other delusions also occur and it can be difficult to distinguish between a true delusion and overvalued ideas in someone with cognitive impairments.

Hallucinations are slightly less common than delusions, and when they occur, they are usually visual. Usually images are of people or animals, but may be striking and complex and rarely people will see complex scenes, often of Lilliputian figures (Ballard et al, 1997a, 1997b). Auditory hallucinations are less common in the early stages but may occur in the later stages of dementia. It is extremely difficult to assess auditory hallucinations. Carers often report that the patient is apparently talking to an invisible person but whether this is a hallucination or not is impossible to decide on many occasions. Visual hallucinations are a key symptom of DLB and PDD (McKeith et al, 2005), when they are often very intense and persistent (Ballard et al, 1997a, 1997b; Ballard et al, 2001) and often accompanied by other psychotic symptoms such as auditory hallucinations, secondary delusions and delusional misidentifications, as well as a cluster of other symptoms which include fluctuating confusion, signs of Parkinsonism, and falls (McKeith et al, 1996; McKeith et al, 2005; Ballard et al, 1997b). Prominent or persistent visual hallucinations in people with mild dementia (Ballard et al, 1999) should always flag DLB as a likely diagnosis.

The frequency of psychosis and agitation is similar in patients with vascular dementia to people with AD, but delusions as well as visual hallucinations are significantly more frequent in DLB (Ballard et al, 1999) and PDD (Aarsland et al, 2001).

Prospective studies demonstrate that hallucinations often resolve over a few months in AD (Ballard et al, 1997a), but delusions and agitation are more persistent (Margallo-Lana et al, 2001). Importantly, 90% of people with dementia develop behavioural problems or psychiatric symptoms at some point during their illness (Ballard and Howard, 2006). These symptoms are frequently distressing for the patients who experience them, are problematic for their caregivers and often precipitate institutional care. Despite the importance of neuropsychiatric symptoms, they remain a major clinical challenge, with no established treatment approaches that are both safe and effective.

Case report

Mrs A and Mrs B lived within a few hundred yards of each other. Both had AD of moderate severity, having been present for 4 years in the case of Mrs A and more than 6 years in the case of Mrs B. Both were under the care of the same specialist team and received home-care support and regular visits from a community psychiatric nurse. Both complained of visitations to their house. Mrs A believed that people were coming through her front door and scampering around her flat. This occurred at any time of day and night and she kept a wooden stick handy to defend herself. She had never seen these people but believed that they stole things from her. As evidence, she led her physician into a dark cupboard and showed him a half-empty carton of washing powder. She believed that these intruders were emptying it. Mrs B on the other hand believed that her intruders came through an upstairs window. Her belief was that someone came into her house and took her money, or sometimes directly from her bank. On closer questioning of Mrs B, it appeared that, in contrast to Mrs A, she did see her intruder and said it was always the same man and sometimes she saw him up a ladder. It turned out that Mrs A was having true delusions but that Mrs B was indeed being visited by her window cleaner who did steal money from her and when seen by Mrs B managed to persuade her to write out cheques for him. The police were informed about Mrs B while Mrs A received pharmacological treatment.

Aetiology of agitation and psychosis

The majority of aetiological studies examining agitation have focused on aggression. From a neurobiological perspective, greater neuronal loss (Forstl et al, 1994), cholinergic deficits (Minger et al, 2000) and altered adrenergic function have been reported as associations of aggression in post-mortem studies (Russo-Neustadt and Cotman, 1997; Sharp et al, 2007). At a clinical level, aggression has been shown to correlate very highly with

psychosis (Aarsland et al, 1996) and the presence of delusions are the best clinical indicator for occurrence of aggressive features (Gilley et al, 1997; Gormley et al, 1998). However, aggression is often situation specific and frequently occurs in response to the environment or some other event, especially those related to personal care (Mintzer and Brawman-Mintzer, 1996).

Psychotic symptoms are probably associated with the severity of the illness (Drevets and Rubin, 1989), seem to occur more often in women than in men (Hirono et al, 1998) and may be more likely in people with hearing difficulties (Ballard et al, 1995). Some evidence points to genetic vulnerability in some individuals associated with specific loss of some neurons or some regions of the brain. For example, both serotonin-receptor-gene (Holmes et al, 1998) and dopamine-receptor-gene (Sweet et al, 1998) polymorphisms have been associated with psychosis in AD. Loss of certain neuronal populations, in particular those of the dorsal raphe nucleus, has been reported in psychosis in AD (Forstl et al, 1994), several studies report an association between delusions and upregulation of muscarinic M1 or M2 receptors in DLB and AD (Ballard et al, 2000b; Lai et al, 2001; Teaktong et al, 2005) and psychosis in general appears to increase in frequency with greater burden of neurofibrillary tangles (Farber et al, 2000). The presence of impaired visual acuity or visual pathology often underlies visual hallucinations in patients with AD (Holroyd 1996; Chapman et al, 1999). In DLB, there is a well-established relationship between visual hallucinations and reduced cholinergic function (Perry et al, 1990; Ballard et al, 2000a, 2000b), but the relationship is less clear in the context of AD (Minger et al, 2000). Although the noradrenergic system has been less studied, one report suggests an association between psychosis and the relative preservation of norepinephrine in the substantia nigra (Zubenko et al, 1991). Functional neuroimaging studies have suggested that hypoperfusion of the left frontal lobes is associated with delusions whereas parietal lobe hypoperfusion is associated with hallucinatory experiences (Kotrla et al, 1995) and hypoperfusion of the occipital cortex has been reported as a specific association of visual hallucinations in DLB (Colloby et al, 2002). There is very little information about the associations of psychosis in people with vascular dementia.

Assessment of agitation and psychosis

Assessment of agitation and psychosis starts with a careful history from an informant. The nature and natural history of the neuropsychiatric symptoms or behavioural disturbance are noted, focusing upon good clinical principles such as When did it start, has it got worse, exactly what occurs? For agitation, the relation between the behavioural disturbance and activities or recent events should be sought. Does the behavioural disturbance only occur when the patient is interacting with another? Did it first start when the patient was admitted to a home? What steps have been taken so far and has there been any change? It is critical to establish the recent health of the patient, and any medication currently or recently taken. The examination should include an observation wherever possible (although this is surprisingly often difficult to achieve) and assessment of the environment before a physical examination for concurrent illness or affective disorder. A key objective is to identify underlying or contributing causes such as delirium, physical illness, pain, affective disturbances, sensory impairments and in the case of behavioural symptoms, concurrent psychosis. Investigations should therefore include a screen for physical illness, especially infection.

Instruments have been developed to assess behavioural disturbance and neuropsychiatric symptoms objectively and reliably; these have enabled research on the causes, effects and management of symptoms and also have an important role in clinical practice, particularly in specialist multidisciplinary care (discussed more fully in chapter 9). Standardised behaviour scales not only measure change reliably but also enable different members of the team to have a commonly agreed baseline assessment on which to build specialist assessments appropriate to their various disciplines. The neuropsychiatric inventory (NPI – Cummings et al, 1994) provides a fairly quick and broad assessment of psychiatric symptoms and behavioural disturbances, and can be complemented with more specialised assessment if needed.

Management of agitation and psychosis

As noted earlier, the first step in management is accurate assessment treatment of any underlying cause of the neuropsychiatric symptom or behavioural disturbance. For example, it goes without saying that if the agitation is because of inadequate analgesia for an arthritic knee, if the wandering is because of increased confusion secondary to concurrent infection or if psychsosis is part of a delirium, then treatment should address these issues before any general management approach is considered.

Psychosocial interventions

In the management of general agitation or specific key behavioural symptoms such as shouting, there are two main psychosocial approaches – formal therapy-based interventions targeted at specific symptoms and more generic psychosocial treatments which aim to increase general well-being by promoting meaningful occupation for the person, by increasing self-expression, improving communication skills and interaction, providing opportunities to enhance personal identity, develop a sense of self-esteem and achievement and provide opportunities to augment psychological interventions with sensory treatment approaches. The most effective psychological approach for addressing specific symptoms, which result in sustained improvement, is behaviour therapy (Livingston et al, 2005). These are individually tailored interventions based on antecedent–behaviour–consequence (ABC) diary assessments (e.g. Moniz-Cook et al, 2001) However, they require skilled assessment and development of the intervention and in practice are often not implemented consistently which reduces their efficacy.

Simple-targeted interventions based on environmental modifications or social interaction can also confer significant benefits (Cohen-Mansfield and Werner, 1997, Cohen-Mansfield et al, 2007) and can be implemented based on a person-centred assessment and often require only brief periods of intervention from caregivers.

Case studies

An elderly man with mild dementia repeatedly asked his wife whether it was dinner time soon. She, thinking this was the best approach, spent much of the day telling him the date, the time, and the weather and placed orientation boards in the living room and kitchen, just as she had seen in day centres she had visited. Whenever he asked if it was nearly dinner time, she took him to one of the boards and tried to orientate him. This caused her to become frustrated and him to become agitated. The situation seemed to be escalating. To try to break the cycle, the doctor in the team reassured her that it was unlikely that continual orientation practice would effect his disease progression and the community nurse persuaded her to remove both the orientation boards. She was encouraged to answer his question and to respond positively when he was correct or to carefully correct him when he was wrong. When he asked whether it was time for dinner it was suggested she reply 'soon, dear', 'quite a while, yet', or ask if he was hungry. He carried on asking but, since his wife had been relieved of the duty of re-orientating him, this repeated questioning became just a behaviour and not a disturbance.

In another example, the community team, over time, became aware that a particular nursing home was the source of a disproportionate number of referrals. These came to all members of the team and were for supposedly different behavioural disturbances. On reflection, however, it seemed that all of the referrals were for patients with advanced dementia who wandered within the home. The layout of the home was such that patients could not wander out of the building and, because the living areas were on different floors to the bedrooms, they rarely interfered with the privacy of other residents. A visit to the home and a short training period showed that a particularly conscientious manager thought that wandering was always a sign of some other problem. When it was explained that this was indeed sometimes the case but that patients with dementia sometimes wander for no apparent reason, the manager and her staff were reassured and the patients were allowed to walk about the home, safely and without causing disturbance.

Changing behaviours by influencing the carer

While the perception of some behaviours can be changed from disturbed to acceptable with education, this is frequently not the case and the behaviour continues to be experienced as problematic. However, working with the carer to change the carer's behaviour can often result in a lessening either of the behaviour or a diminishing of its impact. The multidisciplinary team has a key role in assessment of the behaviour of the patient, the immediate antecedent, and the response of carers. An intervention should be tailored to the individual carer and patient and designed either to remove the antecedents or to change the carer response. However, we find that one small intervention is more useful than almost any other – advising the carer to leave the patient for a short while if behavioural disturbance starts. Understandably, carers are reluctant to leave a demented person, especially if they are agitated or disturbed. However, when the behavioural disturbance results from an intervention made by the carer during a care task – washing or dressing, for example – this is often the only step needed to lessen the behavioural disturbance to manageable levels. We reassure the carer that as long as the patient is safe, then walking away and returning a few minutes later is not only acceptable but of benefit to both, and that this simple act is sometimes the most important thing a dementia team can do.

Equally important, but often harder to address, is the need of the person with dementia for activity. A pleasurable or absorbing activity can greatly lessen behavioural disturbance. While activities as varied as cooking, art and crafts and music can be done easily in an institutional setting, it is important not to underestimate just how difficult it can be for a carer to instigate.

Changing the environment

Persons with dementia are often highly responsive to the environment they find themselves in. In general terms, the environment should be safe and familiar and unnecessary changes should be resisted. Safety is particularly important to allow a carer to leave a disturbed patient for a little while without worrying. An occupational-therapy assessment of a home environment can be

particularly useful to identify potential dangers and to instigate specific measures, such as locking away dangerous tools or kitchen implements. Wandering can be made safe by restricting a person to a specific area but this entails the constant attention to balancing personal autonomy and managing behaviour.

Pharmacotherapy

Most treatment studies have grouped together a variety of neuropsychiatric and behavioural symptoms (usually psychosis, agitation, sleep, appetite changes, elation and apathy); this may be problematic, as it is far from clear that they are underpinned by the same neurochemical or neuropathologial changes. If good clinical management principles are followed, pharmacological intervention should be necessary for only a modest proportion of people with dementia experiencing neuropsychiatric or behavioural symptoms.

Antipsychotics

Antipsychotics are widely used as the first-line pharmacological approach to treat neuropsychiatric and behavioural symptoms in people with dementia. Since 1995, 18 placebo-controlled trials examined the efficacy of atypical neuroleptics over 6 to 12 weeks in people with AD (Ballard and Howard, 2006). The best evidence base is for risperidone, where there are five published trials indicating a modest but significant improvement in aggression compared to placebo, with a larger effect size at 2 mg/day, but only marginal evidence of benefit for psychosis and no benefit for other symptoms of agitation such as wandering and shouting (Ballard and Howard, 2006). The efficacy of other agents has not been established from the trials so far conducted (Ballard and Howard, 2006). Given that in the United States and Europe, 40% to 60% of people with dementia residing in care facilities are prescribed neuroleptics (e.g. Margallo-Lana et al, 2001), for median periods of greater than a year (Ballard et al, 2004; Cohen-Mansfield et al, 1999), an additional pivotal question is whether longer term therapy with atypical neuroleptics confers any treatment benefit. There are only 3 placebo-controlled trials of a neuroleptic for the treatment of behavioural and psychiatric symptoms over periods of 6 to 12 months, none showing clinically meaningful benefit with longer term therapy (Ballard et al, 2005; Schneider et al, 2006 – CATIE; Ballard et al, 2008 – DART). It should be noted that many of these studies have excluded the people with the most severe behavioural and psychiatric symptoms, who from clinical experience may have a more favourable treatment response. The evidence base is, however, extremely important in emphasising the limited benefits in people with mild-to-moderate symptoms and the lack of evidence of ongoing benefit from continued treatment.

Any beneficial effects of atypical neuroleptics in people with AD must be weighed against the adverse effects, which from recent meta-analyses include parkinsonism, sedation, oedema, chest infections, stroke (odds ratio [OR] 2.5–3) and mortality (OR 1.5–1.7) (e.g. CSM, 2004; FDA, 2005; Schneider et al, 2005; Ballard and Howard, 2006). Emerging evidence has also highlighted accelerated cognitive decline as an important potential consequence of neuroleptics (McShane et al, 1997; Ballard et al, 2005). A meta-analysis has confirmed this observation, indicating 0.7 of an Mini mental state examination point greater decline over 6 to 12 weeks in neuroleptic-treated patients compared to those treated with placebo, which appears modest but represents a doubling in the expected rate of cognitive deterioration over this period.

In the face of this evidence, it is difficult to disagree with the conclusions of the CATIE study (Schneider et al, 2006), suggesting that the very modest benefits of treatment do not outweigh the risks, other than in people with severe symptoms that are resulting in tangible risk or extreme distress and which have not responded to other treatment approaches. It is also clear that even in such circumstances where pharmacotherapy with atypical antipsychotics is indicated, this should be used as an opportunity to review the care plan and instigate other treatment approaches with a view to discontinuing atypical antipsychotics after 3 months for most individuals.

Are there pharmacological alternatives to neuroleptics? Other candidate pharmacological treatments include the anticonvulsants carbamazepine and sodium valproate and the antidepressants trazodone and citalopram. Of these the best evidence is for carbamazepine, which has been shown to be significantly better than placebo for the treatment of agitation in several small placebo-controlled trials (e.g. Tariot et al, 1998), although there is limited information pertaining to adverse events and long-term safety in people with dementia for any of these agents. A Cochrane review concluded that sodium valproate was only effective at higher doses that were associated with unacceptable side effects (Lonergan and Luxenberg, 2007). Open and crossover trials have indicated some potential benefits of trazodone in treating agitation (Sultzer et al, 1997), although the results of double-blind, placebo-controlled trials have been disappointing (Teri et al, 2000). Citalopram was associated in the improvement of a number of behavioural and psychiatric symptoms in a double-blind, placebo-controlled trial (Nyth and Gottfries, 1990) and a small recent double-blind study indicated equivalent efficacy to risperidone (Pollock et al, 2007).

An early systematic review and meta-analysis (Trinh et al, 2003) concluded that cholinesterase inhibitors

have a modest beneficial effect in the treatment of neuropsychiatric and behavioural symptoms, supported by the finding of subsequent Cochrane reviews of the individual cholinesterase inhibitors for the treatment of AD (Birks et al, 2007; Birks and Harvey, 2007; Loy and Schneider, 2007). However, it should, be noted that neuropsychiatric symptoms were only evaluated in a subset of studies, changes in individual symptoms were not evaluated, the majority of participants did not have clinically significant neuropsychiatric and behavioural symptoms and the treatment benefits compared to placebo were identified after 6 months of therapy. Three recent studies examining people with significant neuropsychiatric and behavioural symptoms have produced contradictory results. In a small randomised trial focusing on people with mild neuropsychiatric symptoms, Holmes et al (2004) reported a significant 5-point advantage of donepezil over placebo on the NPI. In a slightly larger study of 93 patients, Ballard et al, focusing specifically on AD patients with clinically significant agitation, reported a non-significant 2-point advantage for rivastigmine compared to placebo over 26 weeks (Ballard et al, 2005). A re-analysis of the data from Feldman and colleagues offers a further important insight, suggesting improvements in mood symptoms and apathy but not agitation with donepezil therapy (Gauthier et al, 2002). In addition, a recent large placebo-controlled trial in AD patients with clinically significant agitation indicated limited benefits in the treatment of agitation after 12 weeks, although cognition did improve (Howard et al, 2007). This literature is difficult to pull together, but it is likely that cholinesterase inhibitors are not going to be a useful short-term treatment for neuropsychiatric and behavioural symptoms. Over 6 months or longer, cholinesterase therapy may well confer benefit, and may reduce the need for other psychotropic medication.

Emerging evidence also indicates that memantine, an NMDA antagonist licensed for the treatment of patients with moderate-to-severe AD, may also be helpful in treating neuropsychiatric symptoms, particularly agitation and aggression (Gauthier et al, 2005; Gauthier et al, 2008; Cummings et al, 2006; Wilcock et al, 2008), with a Cochrane review (McShane et al, 1997) suggesting an effect size in the treatment of neuropsychiatric symptoms similar to that reported in a previous Cochrane review of atypical antipsychotics (Ballard and Howard, 2006) seen with atypical antipsychotics. This is a potentially exciting development, especially as the largest improvement appears to be in symptoms of agitation (Wilcock et al, 2008) and possibly explained by memantine action on NMDA receptors in frontal and cingular cortices, as well as effects on tau phosphorylation (Francis, 2009). However, these data are based on retrospective post hoc analyses and the level of agitation in study participants was modest.

Prospective studies in people with more severe clinically significant agitation are required to determine the place of memantine for the treatment of these symptoms. Given the excellent safety profile of memantine, there is however a strong case for using memantine as a first-line pharmacological treatment for agitation given the uncertainties and risks of other treatment approaches.

Are there alternative therapies for agitation? An increasing number of studies indicate that alternative therapeutic approaches may also provide useful treatment options. The best-studied intervention is aromatherapy. Placebo-controlled trials have been published, each reporting a significant beneficial effect on agitation compared to placebo, with almost complete compliance and minimal side effects (Burns et al, 2002). Lemon balm (Melissa officinalis) or lavender (Lavandula officinalis) oil are the two active agents, which are delivered either by inhalation or skin application. Explanations for the efficacy of aromatherapy range from subjective psychological effects to a direct biological action. The latter could be mediated through active terpenes (key chemical constituents of the aromatherapy oils), which modulate neurotransmitter actions, crossing the blood–brain barrier easily because of their lipophilic properties. Developments of trials in this area will include the use of observational behavioural measures as the primary outcome variable and extend precautions to ensure that the rater is blind (or, in this case, has induced anosmia); and mechanistic studies are essential to maximise the potential therapeutic benefits. Benefits have also been reported with personalised music (Gerdner, 2005, Cohen-Mansfield and Werner 1997).

Conclusion

The current chapter has emphasised the frequency and importance of neuropsychiatric and behavioural symptoms in people with AD, highlighted important aspects of assessment and discussed key treatment issues about the most common symptoms of depression, agitation, psychosis and agitation. Good clinical management relies upon thorough evaluation, the treatment of underlying and contributing causes and a comprehensive approach to general management with an emphasis on non-pharmacological approaches and the restrained and cautious use of pharmacotherapy for severe symptoms associated with risk and marked distress. Sleep disturbances will be discussed in chapter 3.

Summary

- Depression is very common in dementia and should be systematically looked for and treated
- Agitation is common and its causes should be looked for in each patient and often can be managed without psychotropic drugs

- Psychosis with or without hallucinations may be alleviated by psychosocial interventions and environmental modifications
- Antipsychotic drugs have limited efficacy in behavioural disturbances associated with dementia and alternative therapeutic approaches should be considered

References

Aarsland D, Ballard C, Larsen JP, McKeith I (2001). A comparative study of psychiatric symptoms in dementia with Lewy bodies and Parkinson's disease with and without dementia. *Int J Geriatric Psychiatry* 16, 528–36.

Aarsland D, Cummings JL, Yenner G, Miller B (1996). Relationship of aggressive behavior to other neuropsychiatric symptoms in patients with Alzheimer's disease. *Am J Psychiatry* 153, 243–7.

Alexopoulos GS, Abrams RC, Young RC, Shamoian CA (1988). Cornell scale for depression in dementia. *Biol Psychiatry* 23, 271–84.

Bains J, Birks JS, Dening TD (2008). Antidepressants for treating depression in dementia. Cochrane Dementia and Cognitive Improvement Group. *Cochrane Database Syst Rev* 1.

Ballard C, Holmes C, McKeith I, et al (1999). Psychiatric morbidity in dementia with Lewy bodies: a prospective clinical and neuropathological comparative study with Alzheimer's disease. *Am J Psychiatry* 156:1039–45.

Ballard C, Howard R (2006). Neuroleptic drugs in dementia: benefits and harm. *Nat Rev Neurosci* 7, 492–500.

Ballard C, Lana MM, Theodoulou M, et al (2008). A Randomised, Blinded, Placebo-Controlled Trial in Dementia Patients Continuing or

Stopping Neuroleptics (The DART-AD Trial) *PLoS Med* 5, 4 e76 doi:10.1371/journal.pmed.0050076.

Ballard C, Margallo-Lana M, Juszczak E, et al (2005). Quetiapine and rivastigmine and cognitive decline in Alzheimer's disease: randomised double blind placebo controlled trial. *BMJ* 330, 874.

Ballard C, McKeith I, Harrison R, et al (1997b). A detailed phenomenological comparison of complex visual hallucinations in dementia with Lewy bodies and Alzheimer's disease. *Int Psychogeriatrics* 9, 381–8.

Ballard C, Neill D, O'Brien J, et al (2000a). Anxiety, depression and psychosis in vascular dementia: prevalence and associations. *J Affective Disorders* 59, 97–106.

Ballard C, O'Brien J, Coope B, et al (1997a). A prospective study of psychotic symptoms in dementia sufferers: psychosis in dementia. *Int Psychogeriatr* 9, 57–64.

Ballard C, Piggott M, Johnson M, et al (2000b). Delusions associated with elevated muscarinic binding in dementia with Lewy bodies. *Annals Neurol* 48, 868–76.

Ballard C, Saad K, Patel A, et al (1995). The prevalence & phenomenology of psychotic symptoms in dementia sufferers. *Int J Geriatr Psychiatry* 10, 477–85.

Ballard CG, O'Brien JT, Swann AG, et al (2001). The natural history of psychosis and depression in dementia with Lewy bodies and Alzheimer's disease: persistence and new cases over 1 year of follow-up. *J Clinical Psychiatry* 62, 46–9.

Ballard CG, Patel A, Solis M, et al (1996). A one-year follow-up study of depression in dementia sufferers. *Br J Psychiatry* 168, 287–91.

Ballard CG, Thomas A, Fossey J, et al (2004) A 3-month, randomized, placebo controlled, neuroleptic discontinuation study in 100 people with dementia: the neuropsychiatric inventory median cutoff is a predictor of clinical outcome. *J Clin Psychiatry* 65, 114–9.

Birks J, Grimley Evans J, Iakovidou V, Tsolaki M (2007). Rivastigmine for Alzheimer's disease. Cochrane Dementia and Cognitive Improvement Group. *Cochrane Database Syst Rev* 3.

Birks JS, Harvey R (2007). Donepezil for dementia due to Alzheimer's disease. Cochrane Dementia and Cognitive Improvement Group. *Cochrane Database Syst Rev* 3.

Brodaty H, Luscombe G (1998). Psychological morbidity in caregivers is associated with depression in patients with dementia. *Alzheimer Dis Assoc Disord* 12, 62–70.

Burke WJ, Dewan V, Wengel SP, et al (1997). The use of selective serotonin reuptake inhibitors for depression and psychosis complicating dementia. *Int J Geriatr Psychiatry* 12, 519–25.

Burns A, Byrne J, Ballard C, Holmes C (2002). Sensory stimulation in dementia. *BMJ* 325, 1312–3.

Burns A, Jacoby R, Levy R (1990a). Psychiatric phenomena in Alzheimer's disease. III: Disorders of mood. *Br J Psychiatry* 157, 81–6.

Burns A, Jacoby R, Levy R (1990b). Psychiatric phenomena in Alzheimer's disease. II: Disorders of perception. *Br J Psychiatry* 157, 76–81.

Burns A, Jacoby R, Levy R (1990c). Psychiatric phenomena in Alzheimer's disease. IV: Disorders of behaviour. *Bri J Psychiatry* 157:86–94.

Cacabelos R, Rodriguez B, Carrera C, et al (1996). APOE-related frequency of cognitive and noncognitive symptoms in dementia. Methods Find. *Exp Clin Pharmacol* 18, 693–706.

Chapman FM, Dickinson J, McKeith I, et al (1999). Association among visual hallucinations, visual acuity, and specific eye pathologies in Alzheimer's disease: treatment implications. *Am J Psychiatry* 156, 1983–5.

Chen CPLH, Alder JT, Bowen DM, et al (1996). Presynaptic serotonergic markers in community-acquired cases of Alzheimer's disease: correlations with depression and neuroleptic medication. J *Neurochem* 66, 1592–98.

Cipriani A, Furukawa TA, Salanti G, et al (2009). Comparative efficacy and acceptability of 12 new-generation antidepressants: a multiple-treatments meta analysis. *Lancet* 373, 746–758.

Cohen-Mansfield J, Libin A, Marx MS (2007). Non-pharmacological treatment of agitation: a controlled trial of systematic individualized intervention. *J Gerontol A Biol Sci Med Sci* 62, 908–16.

Cohen-Mansfield J, Lipson S, Werner P, et al (1999). Withdrawal of haloperidol, thioridazine, and lorazepam in the nursing home: a controlled, double-blind study. *Arch Int Med* 159, 1733–40.

Cohen-Mansfield J, Werner P (1997). Management of verbally disruptive behaviors in nursing home residents. *J Gerontol A Biol Sci Med Sci* 52, 369–77.

Colloby SJ, Fenwick JD, Williams ED, et al (2002). A comparison of (99 m)Tc-HMPAO SPET changes in dementia with Lewy bodies and Alzheimer's disease using statistical parametric mapping. *Eur J Nuclear Med Mol Imaging* 29, 615–22.

Committee for the Safety of Medicines. Atypical antipsychotic drugs and stroke, 9 March 2004.

Cummings JL, Mega M, Gray K, et al (1994). The neuropsychiatric inventory:comprehensive assessment of psychopathology in dementia. *Neurol* 44, 2308–14.

Cummings JL, Schneider E, Tariot PN, et al (2006) Behavioural effects of memantine in Alzheimer's disease patients receiving donepezil treatment. *Neurol* 67, 57–63.

Devanand DP, Sano M, Tang MX, et al (1996). Depressed mood and the incidence of Alzheimer's disease in the elderly living in the community. *Arch Gen Psychiatry* 53, 175–82.

Donaldson C, Tarrier N, Burns A (1998). Determinants of carer stress in Alzheimer's disease. *Int J Geriatr Psychiatry* 13, 248–56.

Drevets WC, Rubin EH (1989). Psychotic symptoms and the longitudinal course of senile dementia of the Alzheimer type. *Biol Psychiatry* 25, 39–48.

Farber NB, Rubin EH, Newcomer JW, et al (2000). Increased neocortical neurofibrillary tangle density in subjects with Alzheimer disease and psychosis. *Arch Gen Psychiatry* 57, 1165–73.

FDA (2005). Deaths with Antipsychotics in Elderly Patients with Behavioral Disturbances. U.S. Food and Drug Administration, *FDA Public Health Advisory, Centre for Drug Evaluation and Research* 13–17.

Fearon M, Donaldson C, Burns A, Tarrier N (1998). Intimacy as a determinant of expressed emotion in carers of people with Alzheimer's disease. *Psychol Med* 28, 1085–90.

Fischer P (1996). The spectrum of depressive pseudo-dementia. *J Neural Transm* 47, 193–203.

Fischer P, Simanyi M, Danielczyk W (1990). Depression in dementia of the Alzheimer type and in multi-infarct dementia. *Am J Psychiatry* 147, 1484–7.

Fitz AG, Teri L (1994). Depression, cognition, and functional ability in patients with Alzheimer's disease. *J Am Geriatr Soc* 42, 186–91.

Forstl H, Burns A, Levy R, Cairns N (1994). Neuropathological correlates of psychotic phenomena in confirmed Alzheimer's disease. *Br J Psychiatry* 165, 53–9.

Forstl H, Burns A, Luthert P, et al (1992). Clinical and neuropathological correlates of depression in Alzheimer's disease. *Psychol Med* 22, 877–84.

Francis PT (2009). Altered Glutamate Neurotransmission and Behaviour in Dementia: Evidence from Studies of Memantine. *Current Molecular Pharmacology* 2, 77–82.

Gauthier S, Feldman H, Hecker J, et al (2002). Donepezil MSAD Study Investigators Group. Efficacy of donepezil on behavioral symptoms in patients with moderate to severe Alzheimer's disease. *Int Psychogeriatr* 14, 389–404.

Gauthier S, Loft H, Cummings J (2008). Improvement in behavioral symptoms in patients with moderate to severe Alzheimer's disease by memantine: a pooled data analysis. *Int J Geriatr Psychiatry* 23, 537–45.

Gauthier S, Wirth Y, Möbius HJ (2005) Effects of memantine on behavioural symptoms in Alzheimer's disease patients: an analysis of the neuropsychiatric inventory (NPI) data of two randomised, controlled studies. *Int J Geriatric Psychiatry* 20, 459–64.

Gerdner LA (2005). Use of individualized music by trained staff and family: translating research into practice. *J Gerontol Nurs* 31, 22–30

Gilley DW, Wilson RS, Beckett LA, Evans DA (1997). Psychotic symptoms and physically aggressive behavior in Alzheimer's disease. *J Am Geriatr Soc* 45, 1074–9.

Godin O, Dufouil C, Maillard P, et al (2008). White matter lesions as a predictor of depression in the elderly: the 3 C-Dijon study. *Biol Psychiatry* 63, 663–9.

Gormley N, Rizwan MR, Lovestone S (1998). Clinical predictors of aggressive behaviour in Alzheimer's disease. *Int J Ger Psychiatry* 13, 109–15.

Gottfries CG, Karlsson I, Nyth AL (1992). Treatment of depression in elderly patients with and without dementia disorders. *Int Clin Psychopharmacol* 6, 55–64.

Hirono N, Mori E, Yasuda M, et al (1998). Factors associated with psychotic symptoms in Alzheimer's disease. *J Neurol Neurosurg Psychiatry* 64, 648–52.

Holmes C, Arranz M, Collier D, et al (2003). Depression in Alzheimer's disease: the effect of serotonin receptor gene variation. *Am J Medical Genetics* Part B, Neuropsychiatric Genetics: the Official Publication of the International Society of Psychiatric Genetics. 119, 40–3.

Holmes C, Arranz MJ, Powell JF, et al (1998). 5-HT2A and 5-HT2C receptor polymorphisms and psychopathology in late onset Alzheimer's disease. *Hum Mol Genet* 7, 1507–9.

Holmes C, Fortenza O, Powell J, Lovestone S (1997). Do neuroleptic drugs hasten cognitive decline in dementia? Carriers of apolipoprotein E e 4 allele seem particularly susceptible to their effects. *BMJ* 314, 1411.

Holmes C, Wilkinson D, Dean C, et al (2004). The efficacy of donepezil in the treatment of neuropsychiatric symptoms in Alzheimer disease. *Neurol* 63, 214–9.

Holroyd S (1996). Visual hallucinations in a geriatric psychiatry clinic: prevalence and associated diagnoses. *J Geriatr Psychiatry Neurol* 9, 171–5.

Hoogendijk WJ, Sommer IE, Pool CW, et al (1999). Lack of association between depression and loss of neurons in the locus coeruleus in Alzheimer disease. *Arch Gen Psychiatry* 56, 45–51.

Howard RJ, Juszczak E, Ballard CG, et al (2007). Donepezil for the treatment of agitation in Alzheimer's disease. *N Engl J Med* 357, 1382–92.

Jorm AF, van Duijn CM, Chandra V, et al (1991). Psychiatric history and related exposures as risk factors for Alzheimer's disease: a collaborative re-analysis of case-control studies (EURODEM Risk Factors Research Group). *Int J Epidemiol* 20, 43–7.

Jost BC, Grossberg GT (1996). The evolution of psychiatric symptoms in Alzheimer's disease: a natural history study. *J Am Geriatr Soc* 44, 1078–81.

Katona CL, Hunter BN, Bray J (1998). A double-blind comparison of the efficacy and safety of paroxetine and imipramine in the treatment of depression with dementia. *Int J Geriatr Psychiatry* 13, 100–8.

Kessing LV, Andersen PK (2004). Does the risk of developing dementia increase with the number of episodes in patients with depressive disorder and in patients with bipolar disorder? *J Neurol Neurosurg Psychiatry* 75, 1662–1666.

Klatka LA, Louis ED, Schiffer RB (1996). Psychiatric features in diffuse Lewy body disease: a clinicopathologic study using Alzheimer's disease and Parkinson's disease comparison groups. *Neurol* 47, 1148–52.

Kotrla KJ, Chacko RC, Harper RG, et al (1995). SPECT findings on psychosis in Alzheimer's disease. *Am J Psychiatry* 152, 1470–75.

Lai MK, Lai OF, Keene J, et al (2001). Psychosis of Alzheimer's disease is associated with elevated muscarinic M2 binding in the cortex. *Neurol* 57, 805–11.

Levy ML, Cummings JL, Fairbanks LA, et al (1996). Longitudinal assessment of symptoms of depression, agitation, and psychosis in 181 patients with Alzheimer's disease. *Am J Psychiatry* 153, 1438–43.

Livingston G, Johnston K, Katona C, et al (2005). Old Age Task Force of the World Federation of Biological Psychiatry. Systematic review of psychological approaches to the management of neuropsychiatric symptoms of dementia. *Am J Psychiatry* 162, 1996–2021.

Lonergan ET, Luxenberg J (2007). Valproate preparations for agitation in dementia. Cochrane Dementia and Cognitive Improvement Group. *Cochrane Database Syst Rev* 3.

Lopez OL, Kamboh MI, Becker JT, et al (1997). The apolipoprotein E epsilon 4 allele is not associated with psychiatric symptoms or extrapyramidal signs in probable Alzheimer's disease. *Neurol* 49, 794–7.

Lovestone S, Hodgson S, Sham P, et al (1996). Familial psychiatric presentation of Huntington's disease. *J Med Genet* 33, 128–31.

Loy C, Schneider L (2007). Galantamine for Alzheimer's disease and mild cognitive impairment. Cochrane Dementia and Cognitive Improvement Group. *Cochrane Database Syst Rev* 3.

Lukovits TG, McDaniel KD (1992). Behavioral disturbance in severe Alzheimer's disease: a comparison of family member and nursing staff reporting. *J Am Geriatr Soc* 40, 891–5.

Lyketsos CG, Baker L, Warren A, et al (1997a). Depression, delusions, and hallucinations in Alzheimer's disease: no relationship to apolipoprotein E genotype. *J Neuropsychiatry Clin Neurosci* 9, 64–7.

Lyketsos CG, Corazzini K, Steele C (1995). Mania in Alzheimer's disease. *J Neuropsychiatry Clin Neurosci* 7, 350–2.

Lyketsos CG, DelCampo L, Steinberg M, et al (2003). Treating depression in Alzheimer disease: efficacy and safety of sertraline therapy, and the benefits of depression reduction: the DIADS. *Arch Gen Psychiatry* 60, 737–46.

Lyketsos CG, Sheppard JM, Steele CD, et al (2000b). Randomized, placebo-controlled, double-blind clinical trial of sertraline in the treatment of depression complicating Alzheimer's disease: initial results from the Depression in Alzheimer's Disease study. *Am J Psychiatry* 157, 1686–9.

Lyketsos CG, Steele C, Baker L, et al (1997b). Major and minor depression in Alzheimer's disease: prevalence and impact. *J Neuropsychiatry Clin Neurosci* 9, 556–61.

Lyketsos CG, Steele C, Galik E, et al (1999). Physical aggression in dementia patients and its relationship to depression. *Am J Psychiatry* 156, 66–71.

Lyketsos CG, Steinberg M, Tschanz JT, et al (2000a). Mental and behavioral disturbances in dementia: findings from the Cache County Study on Memory in Aging. *Am J Psychiatry* 157, 708–14.

Margallo-Lana M, Swann A, O'Brien J, et al (2001). Prevalence and pharmacological management of behavioural and psychological symptoms amongst dementia sufferers living in care environments. *Int J Geriatr Psychiatry* 16, 39–44

McKeith IG, Dickson DW, Lowe J, et al (2005). Diagnosis and management of dementia with Lewy bodies: third report of the DLB Consortium. *Neurology* 65, 1863–72.

McKeith IG, Galasko D, Kosaka K, et al (1996). Consensus guidelines for the clinical and pathologic diagnosis of dementia with Lewy bodies (DLB): report of the consortium on DLB international workshop. *Neurology* 47, 1113–24.

McShane R, Keene J, Gedling K, Fairburn C, Jacoby R, Hope T (1997). Do neuroleptic drugs hasten cognitive decline in dementia? Prospective study with necropsy follow up. *BMJ* 314, 266–70.

Migliorelli R, Tesón A, Sabe L, Petracchi M, Leiguarda R, Starkstein SE (1995). Prevalence and correlates of dysthymia and major depression among patients with Alzheimer's disease. *Am J Psychiatry* 152, 37–44.

Minger SL, Esiri MM, McDonald B, et al (2000). Cholinergic deficits contribute to behavioral disturbance in patients with dementia. *Neurology* 55, 1460–7.

Mintzer JE, Brawman Mintzer O (1996). Agitation as a possible expression of generalized anxiety disorder in demented elderly patients: toward a treatment approach. *J Clin Psychiatry* 57(suppl), 55–63.

Moniz-Cook E, Woods RT, Richards K (2001). Functional analysis of challenging behaviour in dementia: the role of superstition. *Int J Geriatr Psychiatry* 16, 45–56.

Nyth AL, Gottfries CG (1990). The clinical efficacy of citalopram in treatment of emotional disturbances in dementia disorders. A Nordic multicentre study. *Br J Psychiatry* 157, 894–901

O'Brien JT (2006). Vascular cognitive impairment. *Am J Geriatr Psychiatry* 14(9), 724–36.

Pearlson GD, Ross CA, Lohr WD, Rovner BW, Chase GA, Folstein MF (1990). Association between family history of affective disorder and the depressive syndrome of Alzheimer's disease. *Am J Psychiatry* 147, 452–6.

Perry EK, Marshall E, Kerwin J, et al (1990). Evidence of a monoaminergic-cholinergic imbalance related to visual hallucinations in Lewy body dementia. *J Neurochem* 55, 1454–6.

Petracca G, Teson A, Chemerinski E, Leguarda R, Starkstein SE (1996). A double-blind placebo-controlled study of clomipramine in depressed patients with Alzheimer's disease. *J Neuropsychiatry Clin Neurosci* 8(3), 270–5.

Pollock BG, Mulsant BH, Rosen J, et al (2007). A double-blind comparison of citalopram and risperidone for the treatment of behavioral and psychotic symptoms associated with dementia. *Am J Geriatr Psychiatry* 15, 942–52.

Reichman WE, Coyne AC (1995). Depressive symptoms in Alzheimer's disease and multi-infarct dementia. *J Geriatr Psychiatry Neurol* 8, 96–9.

Reifler BV, Teri L, Raskind M, et al (1989). Double-blind trial of imipramine in Alzheimer's disease patients with and without depression. *Am J Psychiatry* 146, 45–9.

Russo-Neustadt A, Cotman CW (1997). Adrenergic receptors in Alzheimer's disease brain: selective increases in the cerebella of aggressive patients. *J Neurosci* 17, 5573–80.

Schneider LS, Dagerman KS, Insel P, et al (2005). Risk of death with atypical antipsychotic drug treatment for dementia: meta-analysis of randomized placebo-controlled trials. *JAMA* 294, 1934–3.

Schneider LS, Tariot PN, Dagerman KS, et al.; CATIE-AD Study Group (2006). Effectiveness of atypical antipsychotic drugs in patients with Alzheimer's disease. *N Engl J Med* 355(15), 1525–38.

Sharp SI, Ballard CG, Chen CP, Francis PT (2007). Aggressive behavior and neuroleptic medication are associated with increased number of alpha1-adrenoceptors in patients with Alzheimer disease. *Am J Geriatr Psychiatry* 15(5), 435–7.

Speck CE, Kukull WA, Brenner DE, et al (1995). History of depression as a risk factor for Alzheimer's disease. *Epidemiology* 6, 366–9.

Starkstein SE, Chemerinski E, Sabe L, et al (1997). Prospective longitudinal study of depression and anosognosia in Alzheimer's disease. *Br J Psychiatry* 171, 47–52.

Starkstein SE, Migliorelli R, Tesón A, et al (1995). Prevalence and clinical correlates of pathological affective display in Alzheimer's disease. *J Neurol Neurosurg Psychiatry* 59, 55–60.

Steffens DC, Plassman BL, Helms MJ, Welsh-Bohmer KA, Saunders AM, Breitner JCS (1997). A twin study of late-onset depression and apolipoprotein E e 4 as risk factors for Alzheimer's disease. *Biol Psychiatry* 41, 851–6.

Strauss ME, Lee MM, DiFilippo JM (1997). Premorbid personality and behavioral symptoms in Alzheimer disease – Some cautions. *Arch Neurol* 54, 257–9.

Sultzer DL, Gray KF, Gunay I, Berisford MA, Mahler ME (1997). A double-blind comparison of trazodone and haloperidol for treatment of agitation in patients with dementia. *Am J Geriatric Psychiatry* 5, 60–9.

Sweet RA, Nimgaonkar VL, Kamboh MI, Lopez OL, Zhang F, DeKosky ST (1998). Dopamine receptor genetic variation, psychosis, and aggression in Alzheimer disease. *Arch Neurol* 55, 1335–40.

Tariot PN, Erb R, Podgorski CA, et al (1998). Efficacy and tolerability of carbamazepine for agitation and aggression in dementia. *Am J Psychiatry* 155, 54–61.

Teaktong T, Piggott MA, McKeith IG, et al (2005). Muscorinic M2 and M4 receptors in anterior cingulate cortex: relation to neuropsychiatric symptoms in dementia with Lewy bodies. *Behav Brain Res* 161, 229–305.

Teri L, Gibbons LE, McCurry SM, et al (2003). Exercise plus behavioral management in patients with Alzheimer disease: a randomized controlled trial. *JAMA* 290, 2015–22.

Teri L, Logsdon RG, Peskind E, et al.; Alzheimer's Disease Cooperative Study (2000). Treatment of agitation in AD: a randomized, placebo-controlled clinical trial. *Neurology* 55, 1271–8.

Teri L, Logsdon RG, Uomoto J, McCurry SM (1997). Behavioral treatment of depression in dementia patients: a controlled clinical trial. *J Gerontol B Psychol Sci Soc Sci* 52, P159–66.

Trinh NH, Hoblyn J, Mohanty S, Yaffe K (2003). Efficacy of cholinesterase inhibitors in the treatment of neuropsychiatric symptoms and functional impairment in Alzheimer disease: a meta-analysis. *JAMA* 289, 210–6.

Verhey FR, Ponds RW, Rozendaal N, Jolles J (1995). Depression, insight, and personality changes in Alzheimer's disease and vascular dementia. *J Geriatr Psychiatry Neurol* 8, 23–7.

Victoroff J, Mack WJ, Nielson KA (1998). Psychiatric complications of dementia: impact on caregivers. *Dementia* 9, 50–5.

Victoroff J, Nielson K, Mungas D (1997). Caregiver and clinician assessment of behavioral disturbances: the California Dementia Behavior Questionnaire. *Int Psychogeriatr* 9, 155–74.

Vida S, Des Rosiers P, Carrier L, Gauthier S (1994). Depression in Alzheimer's disease: receiver operating characteristic analysis of the cornell scale for depression in dementia and the hamilton depression scale. *J Geriatr Psychiatry Neurol* 7, 159–62.

Vitaliano PP, Young HM, Russo J, Romano J, Magana-Amato A (1993). Does expressed emotion in spouses predict subsequent problems among care recipients with Alzheimer's disease? *J Gerontol* 48, P202–9.

Wilcock GK, Ballard CG, Cooper JA, Loft H (2008). Memantine for agitation/aggression and psychosis in moderately severe to severe Alzheimer's disease: a pooled analysis of 3 studies. *J Clin Psychiatry.* 69, 341–8.

Wragg RE, Jeste DV (1988). Neuroleptics and alternative treatments: management of behavioral symptoms and psychosis in Alzheimer's disease and related conditions. *Psychiatr Clin North Am* 11, 195–213.

Zubenko GS, Moossy J, Martinez AJ, et al (1991). Neuropathologic and neurochemical correlates of psychosis in primary dementia. *Arch Neurol* 48, 619–24.

Zubenko GS, Rosen J, Sweet RA, Mulsant BH, Rifai AH (1992). Impact of psychiatric hospitalization on behavioral complications of Alzheimer's disease. *Am J Psychiatry* 149, 1484–91.

Sleep disturbances

'Doctor, he gets up in the middle of the night and wants to go to work'

Although there are those who seem to survive, or even thrive, on little sleep, for most of us sleep is a welcomed and much-needed end to the day. Undoubtedly the amount of sleep needed changes with age and the elderly sleep less than the young. However, despite a reduced need for sleep with late age, sleep-pattern disturbances common in dementia are stressful both to patients and their carers and present a common management problem.

Sleep consists of five stages, stage 1 (a transitionary phase) leading to stage 2, that of light sleep, characterized by phasic changes on EEG. Stages 3 and 4 are periods of deep sleep with EEG slow waves (slow wave sleep [SWS]), whereas stage 5 is that of rapid desynchronised eye movements (REM). In younger adults, stage 2 occupies approximately half of total sleep time (stages 3 and 4 together occupy 20% and stage 5 or REM sleep occupies 25%). This pattern changes with age, and stage 1 sleep periods increase at the expense of stages 3 and 4. In the very elderly, stage 5 or REM sleep is also decreased. The causes of the changes in sleep pattern with ageing are not fully known. The amount of sleep needed is almost certainly related to extrinsic factors such as the amount of activity undertaken but also to intrinsic cerebral factors. Many physical illnesses also affect sleep, such as prostatism, chest disease, muscular skeletal pain and use of alcohol and caffeine. The physical causes of sleep disturbance are all common in the elderly. However, although sleep patterns do change with age, these changes are more frequent and severe in Alzheimer's disease (AD).

Sleep disturbance

Surveys of patients with AD in a hospital setting and in the community have emphasised the degree of disturbance of sleep accompanying dementia. Rates vary from 67% of patients with some sleep disturbance (Cacabelos et al, 1996) to 20% or less (Cooper et al, 1990). One long-term study of nursing-staff observations over 12 to 18 months found that 24% of nights of AD patients in hospital were disturbed (Bliwise et al, 1995).

Although sleep is disturbed early in the disease process, most of the initial changes are exaggerated responses normally seen in ageing. Most importantly, REM or stage 5 sleep is lost only late in disease progression (Grothe et al, 1998; Vitiello and Prinz, 1989). Early in the course of the disease, activity at night increases and the amplitude of the activity/rest cycle is lower (Satlin et al, 1995). Because activity and wakefulness at night increases, the amount of

stage 1 sleep increases at the expense of deep stage 3/4 sleep (Martin et al, 1986; Prinz et al, 1982a; Vitiello and Prinz, 1989). Later in the disease progression, REM sleep is lost and some studies have reported an increased latency period until REM sleep (Montplaisir et al, 1995; Prinz et al, 1982b). Sleep disturbances such as these are not limited to AD; however, some evidence suggests that the sleep disturbance of vascular dementia can be as severe, or indeed worse, than that found in AD. Measures of both the amount of REM sleep and REM latency, however, may make it possible to distinguish between depression and dementia (Dykierek et al, 1998; Vitiello et al, 1984).

The pathogenesis of sleep disturbance in AD is not understood, although there is evidence to suggest that cholinergic loss is largely the cause (Montplaisir et al, 1995). Although a complex phenomenon, the control of sleep is to a large extent under cholinergic regulation (Riemann et al, 1994). REM sleep itself is clearly under direct control of cholinergic neurones, in particular, the cholinergic tracts running from brainstem nuclei (Everitt and Robbins, 1997); although cerebral mapping of sleep centres with retrograde transport of tagged markers of the cholinergic system have identified other cholinergic pathways and indeed non-cholinergic influence on REM sleep in the cat (Quattrochi et al, 1998). As cholinergic neurones are lost in AD, this is likely to affect sleep over and above the normal changes of ageing and it is almost certainly the loss of cholinergic projection from the nucleus basalis of Meynert that is responsible for loss of REM sleep in moderate dementia. However, in AD, other evidence suggests a more profound disturbance of circadian rhythms in addition to this loss of regulation of sleep architecture. A subgroup of AD patients appear to have impaired synchronisation of core body temperature and circadian cycles (Satlin et al, 1995). Disturbance of the normal circadian rhythms of the hypothalamic pituitary axis is altered in AD (Martignoni et al, 1990; Suemaru et al, 1991; Wallin et al, 1991).

Circadian rhythm control, the biological clock, is located in the suprachiasmatic nucleus and lesions within this small structure can cause complete disruption of the normal wake/sleep cycle. In AD, loss of circadian rhythms is manifested by increased napping during the day and quite possibly also the phenomenon of sundowning whereby behavioural disturbance is exacerbated in the latter part of the day. The control of circadian rhythm by the suprachiasmatic nucleus (SCN) has been shown, in animal studies, to be closely linked to the external light/dark cycle – a process of synchronisation known as N training. In patients with AD, the degree of night-time activity was shown in one study to change according to the season, becoming worse as the days grew longer (Van Someren et al, 1996).

The reason why SCN control of circadian rhythm is altered in AD is unclear but may not be directly due to neuronal loss. Transplantation of transgenic cells overexpressing the amyloid peptide to the SCN of rats caused disruption of circadian rhythm (Tate et al, 1992). Direct evidence of SCN-function abnormalities in AD comes from studies showing altered melatonin rhythms in some, but not all, patients (Uchida et al, 1996).

Sleep disturbance in AD may result from loss of cholinergic influence over REM sleep and altered SCN regulation of circadian rhythms. As may be expected, if there is a direct relation between neuronal loss and sleep disturbance, loss of normal sleep architecture tends to be more severe in those with more severe disease (Bliwise et al, 1995; Ancoli-Israel et al, 1997). The observation that sleep disturbance also correlates with daytime behavioural disturbance (Rebok et al, 1991) may reflect the idea that cholinergic projections to the thalamus regulate sleep disturbance, while cholinergic projections to midbrain dopamine neurons are responsible for behavioural disturbance in AD (Everitt and Robbins, 1997). Loss of nucleus basalis Meynert neurons would give rise to both simultaneously. However, in addition to sleep disturbance resulting from the pathogenesis of AD, changes in sleep may occur commonly in AD because of extrinsic factors. Physical causes of insomnia are common, particularly with increasing frailty, and the decreased activity inherent in moderate AD contributes to increased activity at night.

Sleep disturbance and carers

Loss of sleep itself is distressing for patients and can be of primary concern to carers. However, loss of sleep is almost always accompanied by altered behaviour during wakefulness at night and this has a substantial impact on carers. It has also been shown that even daytime behavioural disturbance is associated with night-time sleeplessness (Rebok et al, 1991). Not surprisingly, sleep disturbance is among the most stressful of behavioural disturbances reported by carers (Donaldson et al, 1998); it is easy to see how loss of sleep in the patient results in loss of sleep in the carer, which will impact on their ability to look after the patient. An escalation can ensue, resulting in a complete loss of morale and breakdown in the home situation.

Persons with AD vary considerably in their behaviours on waking. Some patients are quiet on waking, although the carer may be aware that they are awake. More commonly, however, the patient on waking, will get up and pace around the home or act as if it is daytime. For this reason, the primary focus of treatment of sleep disturbance, at least when the patient lives at home, should be to ensure that the carer gets an adequate night's sleep.

Case history

A 72-year-old man with moderate AD was very well cared for at home by his wife. Other than attending a day centre twice a week, the couple used no other services and indeed no other facilities were deemed necessary. It was a surprise, therefore, when he and his wife were brought by relatives to an emergency admission unit. It appeared that he had begun to wake at night and would get up and attempt to make his wife breakfast. Fearing he would come to some harm, she had taken to sleeping in his bedroom, so she would wake when he did. Not surprisingly, she too began to suffer from severe loss of sleep. When relatives came to visit they found both of them unkempt and distressed. In response, a night-time sitter was arranged for one day a week and the carer encouraged to take whatever opportunity she could to catch up on her sleep during the time the patient was at the day centre. Just 3 weeks later she had returned to her former highly competent and organised state and the crisis had passed.

Non-pharmacological interventions

Before considering specific management approaches, it is important to ensure that expectations are realistic. Most older people sleep for 6 hours or less a night, and that pattern is often distributed more evenly over 24 hours in people with dementia. Particularly in care homes and nursing homes, framing a sleep pattern as 'abnormal' when an individual does not sleep from 8 PM to 8 AM requires education as to the expected sleep patterns in these individuals. Within care settings, this may well need to be linked to 'person-centered' practices including, enabling people to choose the time at which they want to go to bed and planning activities and staffing levels to meet the 24-hour active needs of residents with dementia (Train et al, 2005). Balancing the needs of the individual with dementia against the needs of the principle carer can be more challenging when someone is living at home.

The first step of managing any problem is taking a detailed history, in this case, to understand the pattern of sleep and any perceived disturbance – when does the patient sleep by day and by night, where do they sleep, what do they do before going to sleep, and what happens on waking during the night? A thorough physical assessment is mandatory – is there evidence of respiratory disease, heart failure, peripheral vascular disease, arthritis, chronic back pain, prostatism, or other causes of sleep disturbance?

Sleep disordered breathing, usually defined as a respiratory disturbance index of greater than 10 events per hour of sleep (Ancoli-Israel et al, 1989), is highly prevalent (84%) in people with dementia and should always be considered as a specific differential diagnosis. Other important considerations in the differential diagnosis include other medical and psychiatric disorders, especially delirium, depression, anxiety and chronic pain; other sleep disorders and parainsomnias (e.g., periodic limb movement disorder, restless legs syndrome, REM sleep Behaviour Disorder (RBD), behavioural manifestations of epileptiform activity). Medication use is high in this population, and many commonly used drugs may be associated with insomnia and/or daytime sleepiness in nursing home populations. (Bliwise et al, 1990, Little et al, 1995, Alessi et al, 1995). In addition, cholinesterase inhibitors may induce insomnia in some individuals (6–14%) (Sramek et al, 2001). Medication should therefore be reassessed, including attention to over-the-counter preparations such as stimulants or nasal decongestants. The amount of activity by day should be assessed, as should the use of alcohol and coffee before bedtime.

Non-pharmacological management of sleep disturbance should always be attempted before drug treatment. The concept of sleep hygiene is useful in managing the sleep disturbance itself. Daytime naps should be prevented wherever possible and activity by day maximised. The relation between daytime activity or mild exercise and increased sleep is preserved in AD. Patients should be encouraged to sleep in a bedroom (not, for example, in a comfortable chair in the living room) and the bedroom should be darkened, peaceful, and used for sleep only. While a small amount of alcohol rarely does harm, excess alcohol use should be prevented. Evening drinks should be warm and milky rather than caffeine enriched. Attention should be paid to mealtimes; many elderly people in congregate settings are given a substantial and heavy meal at midday and this can induce a soporific state in the afternoon. A light luncheon and a main meal early in the evening (some hours before bedtime) can be helpful for some patients. Evidence exists that sleep patterns can be rectified by interventions such as increased exercise and social contact (Okawa et al, 1991). Sleep hygiene measures do work if enforced rigorously, especially is supported by a carer 'work diary' describing the interventions and their impact.

A novel non-pharmacological approach that appears promising is the use of bright light to attempt resynchronising circadian rhythms. From the discussion of the biology of sleep, it is apparent that this can only rectify one part of the regulation of sleep but, nonetheless, some evidence has accumulated that, at least for some patients, sleep disturbance is reduced with bright light (Campbell et al, 1988; Satlin et al, 1992; Van Someren et al, 1993; Van Someren et al, 1997, evidence reviewed by Burns et al, 2002; Ancoli-Israel et al, 2003). There is some preliminary evidence that metatonin may improve sleep and diurnal activity patterns in persons with dementia (Dowling et al, 2008). Lavender, applied as an aromatherapy oil, may also help promote sleep (Burns et al, 2002),

and may provide a welcomed and side-effect free alternative to hypnotics for some patients.

Pharmacological interventions

There is no effective, unproblematical pharmacotherapy for sleep disturbance in AD. Benzodiazepines are, not surprisingly, the most commonly prescribed drugs. However, there is little evidence for effectiveness in AD (McCarten et al, 1995) and much evidence of substantial side effects, including a markedly increased risk of falls and increased confusion. If benzodiazepines must be used, then the short-acting compounds are preferable to avoid hangover sedation. However, an ultrashort-acting benzodiazepine, triazolam, withdrawn in some countries because of side effects, had no beneficial effects in AD sleep disturbance (McCarten et al, 1995). Even where effective for increasing sleep, benzodiazepines can only be a very short-term solution for occasional use in crises – to give a carer a short break from sleep disturbance, for example. Longer use will lead to tolerance, with a loss of effectiveness, accompanied by dependence.

Sedating antidepressants can be useful, particularly if there is a suggestion that sleeplessness is accompanying altered mood. Trazodone, for example, is highly sedating and can be effective in reducing symptoms of depression and inducing sleep at the same time. Some patients become highly disturbed at night and other pharmacological interventions are necessary as for similar behavioural disturbance by day.

Because increasing cholinergic neurotransmission increases activity and energy, cholinesterases inhibitors would be expected to have an adverse effect on sleep. One of the most commonly reported subjective effects of dementia treatments is that the person seems more 'alive' and 'awake'. Fortunately, this does not appear to extend to being awake at night. Trials of cholinesterases inhibitors have shown either no change (Holsboer-Trachsler et al, 1993) or, possibly, even a small beneficial effect on sleep disturbance (Holsboer-Trachsler et al, 1993; Gillman, 1997).

REM sleep behaviour disorder

REM sleep behaviour disorder (RBD) merits specific consideration because of the potential association with the presentation of specific dementias. RBD is characterized by complex behaviour and a loss of skeletal muscle atonia during REM sleep. This parasomnia, first described by Schenck and colleagues (Schenck et al, 1986) is characterized by movements of the limbs or body associated with dream mentation, dreams that appear to be acted out and sleep behaviour that disrupts sleep continuity. Patients often recall aggressive or violent dreams and sometimes injure their bed partner or themselves during episodes of RBD.

The loss of voluntary muscle atonia during REM sleep is a typical finding in polysomnography. RBD has a population frequency of 0.5%, but is more frequent in the 6th and 7th decade, and in men (Schenck and Mahowald, 2002). Clinical reports indicate that RBD is frequently associated with LB disease but rarely with other neurodegenerative disorders (Boeve et al, 2003).

Of particular importance with respect to the treatment of patients with dementia, several retrospective reports indicate that the clinical symptoms of RBD precede the onset of neurological disease such as Parkinson's disease (PD) (Olson et al, 2000) and dementia with Lewy bodies (DLB) (Boeve et al, 1998) by 1 to 7 years. This body of work is supported by prospective studies. For example, Schenck et al (1996) reported that 11 of 29 (38%) people with RBD developed a parkinsonian syndrome 7 years after onset of RBD (4 years of follow-up). In a second recent prospective study, Iranzo and coworkers assessed survivors of 44 patients with idiopathic RBD who had been diagnosed 5 years earlier. Forty-five percent had developed a neurological disorder, usually of the α-synuclein type, such as PD or DLB, based on clinical evaluation (Iranzo et al, 2006). The findings are also consistent with the current autopsy literature, which indicates that RBD is underpinned by α-synuclein pathology in all the cases so far reported (as reviewed in Boeve et al, 2007). RBD is a clinical syndrome in its own right. Thus patients presenting with early cognitive impairment associated with RBD are very likely to develop DLB rather than AD.

Managing sleep disturbance: conclusions

Sleep disturbance in AD starts with exaggerations of the sleep loss normal in late life but accelerates to include loss of REM sleep and altered circadian rhythms. As well as neurodegenerative causes of such sleep loss, there are many physical causes of sleep loss common in AD patients. Management of sleep disturbance starts with a full and comprehensive assessment. Education and information to carers is sometimes sufficient and always necessary. At times carers worry about decreased sleep in the person they are caring for even if this is causing neither them nor the patient a problem. If the patient loses sleep but does not disturb the carer, then no further treatment may be necessary. If the disturbed behaviour during wakefulness can be managed in some other way, then managing the sleep disturbance itself may not be necessary. However, if the sleep disturbance itself is to be treated, then sleep-hygiene approaches and increasing activity by day are most important and should be attempted first. Pharmacological management alone is rarely effective in the long term.

Sleep disturbance can persist despite aggressive assessment and intervention. In these situations, the impact of the disturbance on carers should be minimised. Night-time sitters should be sought and respite periods in residential settings arranged. Although unsatisfactory in many ways, carers can catch up with sleep during the day when the patient attends a day centre. For some patients and their carers, however, persistent and severe sleep disturbance is the main reason for entry into long-term care.

Summary

- Sleep disturbance is an early and common symptom in AD.
- Early in the disease process light (stage 1) sleep displaces deep (stage 3 and 4) sleep; later in the disease process REM (dream) sleep is lost.
- While the cause of sleep loss in AD is not fully understood, increasing evidence point to loss of cholinergic neurons and loss of control of circadian rhythms.
- Sleep disturbance increases daytime and night-time behavioural disturbance and has a profound effect on carers.
- Treatment of sleep disturbance is one of the most productive interventions for patients with AD and their carers – behavioural management being the mainstay of treatment.
- Behavioural management consists predominantly of good sleep hygiene – changing the behaviour so that

night and bedrooms are for sleeping whereas day and living rooms and outside are for wakefulness and energy expenditure.

- Pharmacological management is always problematical and rarely efficacious when used alone.

References

Alessi CA, Schnelle JF, Traub S, Ouslander JG (1995). Psychotropic medications in incontinent nursing home residents: association with sleep and bed mobility. *J Am Geriatr Soc* 43, 788–92.

Ancoli-Israel S, Klauber MR, Jones DW, et al (1997). Variations in circadian rhythms of activity, sleep, and light exposure related to dementia in nursing-home patients. *Sleep* 20, 18–23.

Ancoli-Israel S, Klauber MR, Kripke DF, et al (1989). Sleep apnea in female patients in a nursing home: increased risk of mortality. *Chest* 96, 1054–8.

Ancoli-Israel S, Martin JL, Gehrman P, et al (2003). Effect of light on agitation in institutionalized patients with severe Alzheimer's disease. *Am J Geriatr Psychiatry* 11, 194–203.

Bliwise DL, Carroll JS, Dement WC (1990). Predictors of observed sleep/wakefulness in residents in long-term care. *J Gerontol A Biol Sci Med Sci* 45, M126–30.

Bliwise DL, Hughes M, McMahon PM, Kutner N (1995). Observed sleep/wakefulness and severity of dementia in an Alzheimer's disease special care unit. *J Gerontol* 50A, M303–6.

Boeve BF, Silber MH, Ferman TJ, et al (1998). REM sleep behavior disorder and degenerative dementia: an association likely reflecting Lewy body disease. *Neurology* 51, 363–70.

Boeve BF, Silber MH, Parisi JE, et al (2003). Synucleinopathy pathology and REM sleep behavior disorder plus dementia or parkinsonism. *Neurology* 61, 40–45.

Boeve BF, Silber MH, Saper CB, et al (2007). Pathophysiology of REM sleep behaviour disorder and relevance to neurodegenerative disease. *Brain* 130(pt 11), 2770–88.

Burns A, Byrne J, Ballard C, Holmes C (2002). Sensory stimulation in dementia. *BMJ* 325, 1312–3.

Cacabelos R, Rodriguez B, Carrera C, et al (1996). APOE-related frequency of cognitive and noncognitive symptoms in dementia. *Methods Find Exp Clin Pharmacol* 18, 693–706.

Campbell SS, Kripke DF, Gillin JC, Hrubovcak JC (1988). Exposure to light in healthy elderly subjects and Alzheimer's patients. *Physiol Behav* 42, 141–4.

Cooper JK, Mungas D, Weiler PG (1990). Relation of cognitive status and abnormal behaviors in Alzheimer's disease. *J Am Geriatr Soc* 38, 867–70.

Donaldson C, Tarrier N, Burns A (1998). Determinants of carer stress in Alzheimer's disease. *Int J Geriatr Psychiatry* 13, 248–56.

Dowling GA, Burr RL, van Someren EJW, et al (2008). Melatonin and bright-light treatment for rest-activity disruption in institutionalized patients with Alzheimer's disease. *J Am Geriatr Soc* 56, 239–246.

Dykierek P, Stadtmuller G, Schramm P, et al (1998). The value of REM sleep parameters in differentiating Alzheimer's disease from old-age depression and normal aging. *J Psychiatr Res* 32, 1–9.

Everitt BJ, Robbins TW (1997). Central cholinergic systems and cognition. *Annu Rev Psychol* 48, 649–84.

Gillman PK (1997). Tacrine for treatment of sleep disturbance in dementia. *J Am Geriatr Soc* 45, 1286.

Grothe DR, Piscitelli SC, Dukoff R, Fullerton T, Sunderland T, Molchan SE (1998). Penetration of tacrine into cerebrospinal fluid in patients with Alzheimer's disease. *J Clin Psychopharmacol* 18, 78–81.

Holsboer-Trachsler E, Hatzinger M, Stohler R, et al (1993). Effects of the novel acetylcholinesterase inhibitor SDZ ENA 713 on sleep in man. *Neuropsychopharmacology* 8, 87–92.

Iranzo A, Molinuevo JL, Santamaria J, et al (2006). Rapid-eye-movement sleep behaviour disorder as an early marker for a neurodegenerative disorder: a descriptive study. *Lancet Neurol* 5, 572–6.

Little JT, Satlin A, Sunderland T, Volicer L (1995). Sundown syndrome in severely demented patients with probable Alzheimer's disease. *J Geriatr Psychiatry Neurol* 8, 103–6.

Martignoni E, Petraglia F, Costa A, Bono G, Genazzani AR, Nappi G (1990). Dementia of the Alzheimer type and hypothalamus-pituitary-adrenocortical axis: changes in cerebrospinal fluid corticotropin releasing factor and plasma cortisol levels. *Acta Neurol Scand* 81, 452–6.

Martin PR, Loewenstein RJ, Kaye WH, Ebert MH, Weingartner H, Gillin JC (1986). Sleep EEG in Korsakoff's psychosis and Alzheimer's disease. *Neurology* 36, 411–14.

McCarten JR, Kovera C, Maddox MK, Cleary JP (1995). Triazolam in Alzheimer's disease: pilot study on sleep and memory effects. *Pharmacol Biochem Behav* 52, 447–52.

Montplaisir J, Petit D, Lorrain D, Gauthier S, Nielsen T (1995). Sleep in Alzheimer's disease: further considerations on the role of brainstem and forebrain cholinergic populations in sleep-wake mechanisms. *Sleep* 18, 145–8.

Okawa M, Mishima K, Hishikawa Y, Hozumi S, Hori H, Takahashi K (1991). Circadian rhythm disorders in sleep-waking and body temperature in elderly patients with dementia and their treatment. *Sleep* 14, 478–85.

Olson EJ, Boeve BF, Silber MH (2000). Rapid eye movement sleep behaviour disorder: demographic, clinical and laboratory findings in 93 cases. *Brain* 123(pt 2), 331–9.

Prinz PN, Peskind ER, Vitaliano PP, et al (1982a). Changes in the sleep and waking EEGs of nondemented and demented elderly subjects. *J Am Geriatr Soc* 30, 86–93.

Prinz PN, Vitaliano PP, Vitiello MV, et al (1982b). Sleep, EEG and mental function changes in senile dementia of the Alzheimer's type. *Neurobiol Aging* 3, 361–70.

Quattrochi J, Datta S, Hobson JA (1998). Cholinergic and non-cholinergic afferents of the caudolateral parabrachial nucleus: a role in the long-term enhancement of rapid eye movement sleep. *Neuroscience* 83, 1123–36.

Rebok GW, Rovner BW, Folstein MF (1991). Sleep disturbance and Alzheimer's disease: relationship to behavioral problems. *Aging Milano* 3, 193–6.

Riemann D, Hohagen F, Bahro M, et al (1994). Cholinergic neurotransmission, REM sleep and depression. *J Psychosom Res* 38(suppl), 15–25.

Satlin A, Volicer L, Ross V, Herz L, Campbell S (1992). Bright light treatment of behavioral and sleep disturbances in patients with Alzheimer's disease. *Am J Psychiatry* 149, 1028–32.

Satlin A, Volicer L, Stopa EG, Harper D (1995). Circadian locomotor activity and core-body temperature rhythms in Alzheimer's disease. *Neurobiol Aging* 16, 765–71.

Schenck CH, Bundlie SR, Ettinger MG, Mahowald MW (1986). Chronic behavioral disorders of human REM sleep: a new category of parasomnia. *Sleep* 9(2), 293–308.

Schenck CH, Bundlie SR, Mahowald MW (1996). Delayed emergence of a parkinsonian disorder in 38% of 29 older men initially diagnosed with idiopathic rapid eye movement sleep behaviour disorder. *Neurology* 43, 388–93.

Schenck CH, Mahowald MW (2002). REM sleep behavior disorder: clinical, developmental, and neuroscience perspectives 16 years after its formal identification in sleep. *Sleep* 25, 120–38

Sramek J, Alexander B, Cutler N (2001). Acetylcholinesterase inhibitors for the treatment of Alzheimer's disease. *Ann Long Term Care* 9–10, 15–22.

Suemaru S, Hashimoto K, Suemaru K, Maeba Y, Matsushita N, Ota Z (1991). Hyperkinesia, plasma corticotropin releasing hormone and ACTH in senile dementia. *Neuroreport* 2, 337–40.

Tate B, Aboody Guterman KS, Morris AM, Walcott EC, Majocha RE, Marotta CA (1992). Disruption of circadian regulation by brain grafts that overexpress Alzheimer beta/A4 amyloid. *Proc Natl Acad Sci U S A* 89, 7090–94.

Train G, Nurock S, Kitchen G, Manela M, Livingston G (2005). A qualitative study of the views of residents with dementia, their relatives and staff about work practice in long-term care settings. *Int Psychogeriatr.* 17, 237–51.

Uchida K, Okamoto N, Ohara K, Morita Y (1996). Daily rhythm of serum melatonin in patients with dementia of the degenerate type. *Brain Res* 717, 154–9.

Van Someren EJ, Kessler A, Mirmiran M, Swaab DF (1997). Indirect bright light improves circadian rest-activity rhythm disturbances in demented patients. *Biol Psychiatry* 41, 955–63.

Van Someren EJ, Mirmiran M, Swaab DF (1993). Non-pharmacological treatment of sleep and wake disturbances in aging and Alzheimer's disease: chronobiological perspectives. *Behav Brain Res* 57, 235–53.

Van Someren EJW, Hagebeuk EEO, Lijzenga C, et al (1996). Circadian rest-activity rhythm disturbances in Alzheimer's disease. *Biol Psychiatry* 40, 259–70.

Vitiello MV, Bokan JA, Kukull WA, Muniz RL, Smallwood RG, Prinz PN (1984). Rapid eye movement sleep measures of Alzheimer's-type dementia patients and optimally healthy aged individuals. *Biol Psychiatry* 19, 721–34.

Vitiello MV, Prinz PN (1989). Alzheimer's disease. Sleep and sleep/wake patterns. *Clin Geriatr Med* 5, 289–99.

Wallin A, Carlsson A, Ekman R, et al (1991). Hypothalamic monoamines and neuropeptides in dementia. *Eur Neuropsychopharmacol* 1, 165–8.

Genetics

4

'Doctor, what is my risk of getting Alzheimer's disease since my mother died of dementia?'

We are often asked this question by persons in their midlife interested in knowing their risk and acting accordingly through lifestyle changes (see chapter 1). These are not unreasonable requests, considering the higher risk associated with one and even more with two affected parents (Jayadev et al, 2008). There is research and clinical interest in the genetic risk of children of persons with AD (Jarvik et al, 2008), and genetics of dementia are part of the considerations in clinical guidelines for primary care practitioners (Hsiung & Sadovnick, 2007).

The short answer is that it depends on the age of onset of the dementia in the mother or father, assuming that the cause was AD: 'before age 60' (early-onset AD) raises the possibility of autosomal dominant mutations with a 50% risk for each offspring; 'beyond age 75' (late-onset AD) vascular risk factors are likely more important than genetics (as far as we know for now!); 'in between these ages' risk genes such as the one regulating apolipoprotein E (APOE) play an important role in the pathophysiology of AD (Davidson et al, 2007).

This chapter will review the current knowledge on genetic testing in AD based on chapter 5 from the 1st edition of *Management of Dementia*, written by Simon Lovestone, with new insight into pharmacogenomics, e.g., how genes can influence response to treatment.

Genetic testing and early-onset AD

Some forms of early-onset dementia are inherited in an autosomal-dominant fashion, although these are relatively uncommon disorders (6 – 7% of all cases of AD). Mutations in one of three genes appear to be responsible for most of these early-onset autosomal-dominant forms of AD (Panel 4.1).

Panel 4.1
Known mutations causing early-onset Alzheimer's disease

- Amyloid precursor protein (APP), on chromosome 21
- Presenilin 1 (PS1), on chromosome 14
- Presenilin 2 (PS2), on chromosome 1

The *APP* gene on chromosome 21 was the first to be identified but has been shown to be the disease gene in no more than 20 families worldwide. The *PS-1* gene on chromosome 14 is responsible for most cases of early-onset familial AD. *PS-2* on chromosome 1, on the other hand, is an extremely rare cause of early-onset AD. The determination of the mutations responsible for the disease in these families has been the most important step forward in the understanding of the molecular pathogenesis of AD and has had real and immediate clinical implications for a few individuals. If a mutation in a family with any one of these disorders is found, diagnosis is confirmed; in cases of diagnostic uncertainty it can help to distinguish one dementia from another (Geldmacher and Whitehouse, 1997). Molecular diagnosis has now become a real possibility. For those families with an early-onset clearly familial dementia, AD and other rare causes of dementias (some types of frontotemporal dementia, Huntington's disease, dentatorubro-pallidoluysian atrophy and a disorder with migraine, brain hemorrhage, and dementia [CADASIL]) can be diagnosed with absolute certainty in life. The genetic test is only useful as positive identification — failure to find a mutation is meaningful only in those cases where it is known that the pathogenic mutation is present in an affected family member. Also, the test only confirms which dementia is present; it is unable to determine whether a dementia is present. Clearly affected individuals possessed the mutation from conception and yet the disorder only starts in adulthood. To detect the disorder in the early stages remains a clinical and at times difficult task. Molecular genetic testing for diagnosis in these autosomal-dominant conditions follows rather than precedes specialist clinical assessment.

Just as in Huntington's disease, finding a mutation responsible for autosomal-dominant AD opens up not only the possibilities of diagnostic testing for affected individuals but also predictive testing for their relatives. Now that specific treatments are available for AD, and because the prognosis of each of the inheritable dementias differs, it is appropriate to search for mutations in all newly diagnosed familial dementias. It is not always straightforward to find the mutations, however, because for the presenilin genes, and to some extent the *tau* gene, mutations are distributed widely throughout the coding and non-coding sequence of the gene. Nonetheless, departments of medical genetics now have an important role in assisting in the diagnostic process and all such families should be referred to these specialist services. Molecular diagnostic testing, even in these unambiguously familial conditions, does carry some ethical and practical consequences for the family. In an autosomal-dominant pedigree, all first-degree relatives are at an a priori 50% risk. The detection of the mutation in an affected family member does not alter this risk and to that extent no additional information regarding likelihood of suffering from the condition follows for other family members. However, determining a mutation is a different type of knowledge than making a clinical diagnosis. For most families finding a mutation will make the diagnosis concrete and underlie or emphasise the risk that, by virtue of their parentage, they are exposed to. This information can be expected to increase anxiety and in clinical practice does seem to, at least for some family members. Furthermore, finding a mutation in affected family members makes possible predictive testing in other, unaffected, family members and even prenatal testing. These are difficult issues and all family members should be involved in the decision to make a molecular genetic diagnosis in their relatives. This step need not involve specialist genetic counselling – not at this stage – but should be seen as the preparatory stage for genetic counselling in the future.

When a disease-causing mutation is detected in an affected family member, predictive testing can be offered to unaffected family members. There are important technical problems that have to be considered by a genetics department. For example, if only one family member is affected and available for testing, then it can be difficult to establish whether a novel mutation is truly causing the disease or whether it is a non-pathogenic mutation. Another important consideration is penetrance. Although most of the mutations described thus far are fully penetrant — that is, they always cause disease — in at least one family non-penetrance has been reported (Rossor et al, 1996). These considerations and

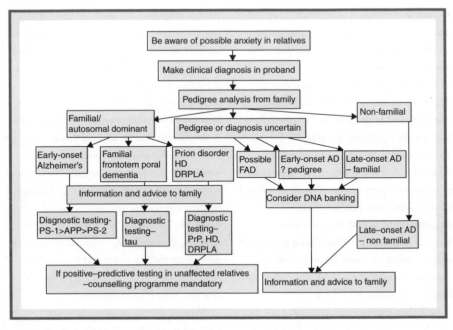

Figure 4.1
Decision making in relation to genetic testing and dementia.

others will be taken into account as advice and information given to family members, but the important point for those clinicians having contact with patients with dementia is that all patients with a clearly familial early-onset dementia should be referred to a specialist genetics department. An algorithm for decision making in relation to genetic testing and dementia is given in Figure 4.1.

Predictive testing for AD should follow guidelines established for Huntington's disease (Burgess, 1994; Lennox et al, 1994). In brief,

testing will be preceded by at least two sessions with two counsellors or geneticists separated by at least 3 months. Some people need more sessions, and follow-up after a test result has been given can be extensive. Such testing should be undertaken only by specialist genetics centres and then with real caution (Scourfield et al, 1997). When conducted in this context, predictive testing has been shown to be safer than feared by many in that most people undergoing testing are less anxious and show less psychological distress at follow-up

(Lawson et al, 1996). However, many individuals choose not to be tested and it may be that a self-selection process operates such that the only people who get tested are those for whom the stress of not knowing is greater than the stress of possibly receiving bad news.

Molecular genetic diagnostic and subsequent predictive testing should only be embarked upon when a dementia is both clearly early in onset and familial. Where the pedigree is not informative — perhaps because the potential carrier-parent died before the age of onset or there are insufficient family members to determine inheritance — then many genetics departments will offer DNA banking. This can be an invaluable service to subsequent generations. DNA from an affected person can be kept virtually in perpetuity, or at least until relatives decide that they want the DNA to be tested or testing becomes feasible (either because a new gene is

discovered or the technology enables more rapid screening for novel mutations). DNA will usually be extracted from a blood sample, although can be obtained by mouth swab and most medical genetics departments will offer DNA banking as a service.

Case study

Two brothers were referred to a specialist clinic for AD genetics by a family doctor. Their family history is shown in Figure 4.2. Their mother died 5 years ago, aged 62, with a dementia that started when she was in her 50s. The dementia was gradual in onset and progression and was accompanied by prominent speech difficulties. Five years after the condition was diagnosed as AD she was almost completely mute. In addition, she was said to have difficulty in walking, frequent

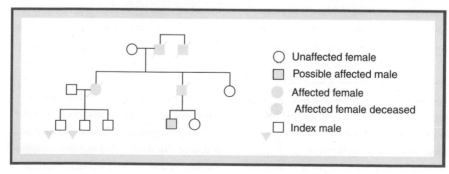

Figure 4.2
Family history of case study.

falls, and a tremor. Her brother was affected by a similar condition but he was said to be irritable and frequently violent towards his wife. Two years before he too received a diagnosis, he had been cautioned by the police for inappropriate sexual behaviour. Very little was known about the maternal grandparent and uncle, but it was believed that both lived their last years in a psychiatric institution and both died in their late 50s or early 60s. A cousin is currently being investigated for a change in behaviour.

The segregation of the disorder in the family suggests autosomal-dominant inheritance, placing the two brothers seeking advice at 50% risk. One of the brothers had pre-teen children and wanted to be able to advise them in due course either that they were at risk of inheriting the condition or that they were not. He felt strongly that when they were of age they should have the opportunity of seeking genetic counselling before contemplating having children. The other brother was newly married and was hoping to have children as soon as possible. However, he felt that if he was going to suffer from the condition he would resolve not to have children because he would not want to subject them to a father becoming demented before they reached adulthood. Both brothers wished at least to consider predictive or pre-symptomatic testing if this were available.

Predictive testing could not be offered to this family because of uncertainty about the disease gene. This family illustrates some of the problems of retrospective diagnosis. Two family members received a lifetime diagnosis of AD by a consultant psychiatrist. However, some elements of the history of their illnesses must raise the suspicion that in fact the disorder was not AD but a similar disorder. In particular, the early speech difficulties and mutism, the disinhibited behavioural pattern and the motor disorder, all point towards the frontotemporal degeneration complex, some of which is associated with motor-neuron disease and some with parkinsonism. Given the multiple possible diagnoses that the responsible gene in the family could have been either the *APP* gene, either of the presenilin genes, the *tau* gene or possibly even the Huntington gene. Alternatively, this could have been one of the autosomal-dominant dementias where a gene has not yet been identified. Had material been available from any of the deceased family members then mutation screening at these loci could have been attempted and, following identification of a disease mutation, it would then have been possible to discover whether or not the two brothers carried the same mutation. If they did, then it would be highly likely that they too would develop the condition; if they did not carry the mutation then, could have been reassured that neither they nor their children would succumb to this particular disorder. Some caution would have been expressed if there was any doubt that the mutation was pathogenic (if it were a novel mutation in the same gene, for example) or if penetrance was not known.

As far as the cousin was concerned, it would have been appropriate to pursue mutation analysis in the absence of other material from an affected member if he was unequivocally suffering from a dementia. In this situation the test would have been diagnostic and not predictive. However, because she was only under investigation for altered behaviour, it was felt inappropriate to conduct diagnostic genetic testing.

These issues are difficult and yet of huge importance to the family. In this family, and in many others, some family members want the information that they do or do not carry a mutation both to settle uncertainty and to make concrete life-planning decisions. Some families and some individuals within all families simply would rather not know. The role of the genetic counsellor is to enable individuals to come to the correct decision for them. Unfortunately, this was not possible in this particular family. Had DNA from a blood sample been kept from the mother, it might well have been.

Genetics of late-onset AD

For late-onset AD the genetics are more complicated, but the issues with respect to counselling more straightforward in that detailed individual genetic counselling is not a prospect for the immediate future. The amount that genetics contributes to personal risk of AD is not entirely clear. However, genetic factors are the largest single risk factor and the only risk factor, other than age, that is consistently identified in all epidemiological studies. Risk of AD increases dramatically over the age of 75 but for those individuals with a family history this increase in risk is even greater. A series of studies have shown that risk increases to 50% or greater in those with an affected first-degree relative by the age of 90 (Breitner, 1994; Huff et al, 1988; Korten et al, 1993).

It has been estimated that one locus, the apolipoprotein E (APOE) gene, contributes about half of the genetic variance (Owen et al, 1994). There are three common variants of APOE in the population coded for by three alleles, namely, B42, B43 and B44. Of these, B43 is the most common, and it has been shown that, relative to B43, the B44 allele increases risk and the B42 allele decreases risk (Roses, 1996). Perhaps risk, although the term often used, is not quite correct, because it appears that the B44 allele has the effect of affecting the chances of suffering from AD by lowering the age at which AD occurs (Meyer et al, 1998). Thus, at any given age those carrying e4 alleles are more likely to develop AD than those not doing so. Each individual has two copies of each gene (or two alleles), one inherited from each parent. It follows that the APOE genotype can be either homozygous (two copies) for B42, B43 or B44, or heterozygous as B42/B43, B43/B44 or B42/B44. Those with two copies of e4 are most at risk, at any given age, and those with two copies of B42 are least at risk. However, the APOE gene is not determinative and some individuals with the B44/B44 genotype reach old age without dementia and many individuals with no e4 alleles are clearly affected.

APOE has been shown to influence the rate of dementia in many diverse populations and has been unequivocally confirmed as the most important genetic influence on late-onset AD. It is likely that many other genes will also contribute to risk either independently or in interaction with APOE. All of these genes may also influence how individuals respond to environmental risk factors as diverse as hypertension, head injury and diet. It has proved difficult to find the other genes associated with late-onset AD.

Many genes have been identified by association studies only to fall by the wayside when other studies fail to confirm the findings. Meta-analysis provides one possible approach to try and make sense of this large volume of literature. A very useful, publicly available, continuously updated database has been created that comprehensively catalogues all genetic association studies relating to Alzheimer's disease (http://www.alzgene.org).

In addition to identifying the e4 allele of APOE and related effects, the meta-analysis has highlighted more than 12 potential Alzheimer's disease susceptibility genes (ACE, CHRNB2, CST3, ESR1, GAPDHS, IDE, MTHFR, NCSTN, PRNP, PSEN1, TF, TFAM and TNF). Most of these confer only a small risk (odds ratio <1.3), but it is likely that there may be numerous similar genes, which may be important at a population level and in further understanding the biology of Alzheimer's disease.

Another promising gene recently identified is the sortilin-related receptor I gene [SORLI] (Rogaeva et al, 2007; Lee et al, 2007). Genome-wide association studies may, in the long run, prove more reliable at identifying regions of chromosomes that are associated with AD and thus point to the genes that alter risk (Li et al, 2008, Waring & Rosenberg, 2008).

Frontotemporal lobar degeneration

Frontotemporal lobar degeneration (FTLD) refers to a group of clinically and pathologically heterogenous disorders leading to early-onset non-Alzheimer's dementia. The main pathological subtypes include patients with ubiquinated inclusions and those with tau-related diagnoses, with clinical presentations that include Frontotemporal Dementia (FTD), semantic dementia, progressive aphasia, FTD with motor neurone disease and FTD with parkinsonism. Approximately half of patients with an FTLD have a family history of a similar disorder (Snowden et al, 1996). The initial crucial discovery was the association between a mutation of the *tau* gene on chromosome 17 and FTD with parkinsonism (Hutton et al, 1998). Subsequently, more than 30 other tau mutations associated with FTLD have been identified, and collectively account for 10% to 20% of FTLD (Rosso et al, 2003). An association has also been reported between FTLD associated with motor neurone disease and an as yet unidentified gene on chromosome 9p (Hosler et al, 2000). More recently, a series of exciting breakthroughs have identified functional mutations of the progranulin gene as the most frequent cause of inherited FTLD (Gass et al, 2006). Progranulin is a peptide growth factor that plays important roles in mediating neuronal development and inflammation. Patients with functional mutations of the progranulin gene often have typical features of FTD, progressive aphasia, and/or parkinsonism, with ubiquitin-positive, tau-negative inclusions at autopsy (Mackenzie et al, 2006). In patients with FTLD, genetic screening of appropriate patients can play an important role in providing an informed prognosis and being

able to offer genetic counselling regarding family risk. In the future, it is likely that specific treatment approaches will be developed targeting specific genetic variants, and that this may also enable more effective treatment of FTLD more generally.

Dementia with Lewy bodies

Patients with dementia with Lewy bodies (DLB) have also an elevated frequency of the apolipoprotein E4 gene (Singleton et al, 2002), which may be associated with a greater burden of concurrent Alzheimer-type pathology in these individuals (Singleton et al, 2002). There has however been little focus upon the specific genetic associations of DLB. Over the last 10 years, there have been major developments in our understanding of the genetics of Parkinson's disease (PD), with various mutations in the synuclein gene (SNCA), the parkin gene and the leucine-rich kinase 2 (LRRK2), all reported as causes of familial PD. The implications of this for our understanding of the genetics of DLB are not yet fully clear, although a recent systematic review of this literature highlighted that 12 out of 24 families with familial PD included individuals with DLB, most frequently associated with SNCA mutations (Kurz et al, 2006).

Clinical consequences of late-onset AD genetics research

It has been suggested that a gene that is associated with late-onset AD such as APOE may be of some clinical use for diagnosis, for prediction, or to assist in management (Roses, 1997). Each of these potential uses is of course complicated by the fact that APOE, and almost certainly this will be true for all other genes associated with AD, neither causes the disease nor entirely protects from the disease. Translation of the effect of APOE into risk is consequently problematical. Take diagnosis, for example, some studies have suggested that diagnostic certainty is increased with APOE genotyping (Roses, 1997; Welsh-Bohmer et al, 1997). The diagnosis of AD can be difficult and is complicated by the fact that AD is by far and away the most common form of dementia, and neuropathological criteria for AD are present in most of those receiving a primary neuropathological diagnosis of some other condition such as vascular dementia. It follows that any diagnostic process, merely by virtue of mathematics, will be very good at determining when AD is present (tossing a coin would be quite good also) but not so good at determining when another condition is also present and quite bad at determining when AD is absent. Indeed, this is exactly what most studies comparing clinical diagnosis to neuropathological diagnosis show — a high

sensitivity and a low specificity. Could APOE genotyping increase the specificity of diagnosis? A very large study examining more than 2000 individuals at necropsy has shown that this is the case combining clinical diagnosis of AD together with APOE genotyping increased specificity of diagnosis at the expense of sensitivity (inevitable as more patients are diagnosed as having some other dementia) for those with an APOE4-positive genotype (Mayeux et al, 1998). However, this was a study conducted in a research setting and whether the same results would be seen in ordinary clinical practice where the range of complicating medical, psychiatric and neurological illnesses is greater is difficult to know. Possibly, a combination of neuroimaging with genotype analysis may have some role in diagnosis (Dubois et al, 2007). The conclusion must be that despite much research, there is no justification for using genetics in routine diagnostic practice at the present time.

Ultimately, the use of APOE genotyping in dementia depends upon how specific the relation is between APOE and AD. As some studies, but not others, have shown an association of APOE with other non-AD dementias such as vascular dementia and Parkinson's disease dementia, the specificity of the relation between AD and APOE is very much open to question. Until these issues are resolved, most groups that have examined the issue think that further data is needed before diagnostic testing using APOE can be recommended in practice.

Predictive testing for AD using the APOE, or any similar gene, is even less likely to find a clinical use than diagnostic testing. Clearly, the fact that APOE only alters risk rather than determining disease status precludes predictive testing of the type done for autosomal-dominant conditions, such as familial early-onset AD or Huntington's disease. When sufficient prospective community-based studies have run their course, it is possible that the degree of risk conferred by APOE or any other gene could be accurately determined. It is possible to envisage a situation where not only could the risk contribution of any one gene be known but also the individual risk of AD based on a combination of genes and environmental factors be determined. Such studies are many years and possibly decades before completion. An early analysis of published studies, however, used an interesting approach that may usefully be replicated when further data from longitudinal population-based studies becomes available. By the use of a Bayesian statistical analysis of lifetime risk at the age of 65 years, it was calculated that the chance of suffering from AD was 15% (Seshadri et al, 1995). Clearly, this is considerably higher than the lifetime risk calculated early in life, because by the age of 65 some of life's risks have been successfully lived through. Adding in APOE knowledge changes the risk to 30% if at least one B44 allele was present and reduced risk to 10% if the individual was free from B44 alleles. The interest in the study comes from the fact that it is at about the age of 65 that individuals begin to worry about getting AD in the future. Few young people are seriously concerned about what may happen in late old age, but as retirement from work and the adjustment to the final period of life (the third age) comes then many begin to wonder what the future holds. We conclude that the change in risk from 15% to either 10% or 30% is too small to be useful. While this is probably true, it may be interesting to learn what 65-year-olds themselves think.

Consensus groups in the United Kingdom and United States have strongly recommended that predictive or susceptibility testing based upon APOE has no place in genetic counselling for AD (Farrer et al, 1995; Medical and Scientific Committee ADI, 1996; Relkin et al, 1996; Hsiung & Sadovnick, 2007).

Finally, genetic risk factors for late-onset AD may influence management of patients with dementia. This is most likely to arise through pharmacogenomics — the possibility that genes may influence response to drug therapies (Poirier & Gauthier, 2008). If a particular genotype at a gene or combination of genotypes were to influence response to cholinesterase inhibitors, for example, then this could influence prescribing habits or policies. Some evidence has suggested that this may indeed be the case with those carrying an APOE4 allele being less likely to respond to this class of compounds (Poirier et al, 1995). However, there might be multiple possible explanations for such an observation and in any case other data is contradictory or fails to support these findings. Nonetheless, such drug targeting by genetic make-up may become an important factor for the future. Response to treatment using disease-modifying drugs may be even more determined by one or more genes (see chapter 7 'Disease-modifying drug treatments').

Genetic testing has little place in the management of dementia of late onset at present. Susceptibility testing is inherently unlikely to ever be possible with a risk-gene as opposed to a determinative-gene, but many clinicians consider that even diagnostic testing is premature at the present time. If genetic variation is shown to alter response to drug therapies, this is the most likely door through which genetic testing will ever be of any practical importance in late-onset AD. Whether such developments would be welcomed by patients, their families or health services remains to be seen.

Summary

- Genetic testing for autosomal-dominant familial early-onset AD is possible at three genes — APP, PS-1 and PS-2.
- Genetic testing can be used in these extremely rare families for diagnosis or for prediction.
- Genetic testing for other dementias is also possible — for example at the tau gene in frontotemporal degeneration with parkinsonism.
- Genetic testing for diagnosis should only be done after discussion with the family; it carries implications for them, as all offspring will be a 50% at risk.
- Predictive testing should follow guidelines established for Huntington's disease.
- AD with an onset before the age of 50 years but without a clear-cut pedigree should be referred to a department of clinical genetics
- Late-onset AD is associated with a risk gene –(APOE) and almost certainly other, yet-to-be discovered risk genes.
- Genetic testing in late-onset AD could be used for diagnosis, prediction, or clinical management. The data thus far, however, does not support either predictive testing or pharmacogenomic applications. Consensus groups have not been convinced by the usefulness of APOE testing for diagnosis.
- Although genetic testing in late-onset AD is not recommended, relatives may still be concerned about inheriting AD genes and should receive appropriate and accurate information.

References

Breitner JCS (1994). Genetic factors. In: Burns A, Levy R, eds. *Dementia*. London, UK: Chapman and Hall; 281–92.

Burgess MM (1994). Ethical issues in genetic testing for Alzheimer's disease: lessons from Huntington's disease. *Alzheimer Dis Assoc Disord* 8, 71–8.

Davidson Y, Gibbons L, Pritchard A, et al (2007). Apolipoprotein E e4 allele frequency and age of onset of Alzheimer's disease. *Dement Geriatr Cogn Disord* 23, 60–6.

Dubois B, Feldman HH, Jacova C, et al (2007). Research criteria for the diagnosis of Alzheimer's disease: revising the NINCDS-ADRDA criteria. *Lancet Neurol* 6, 734–46.

Farrer LA, Brin MF, Elsas L, et al (1995). Statement on use of apolipoprotein E testing for Alzheimer disease. *JAMA* 274, 1627–9.

Gass J, Cannon A, Mackenzie IR, et al (2006). Mutations in progranulin are a major cause of ubiquitin-positive frontotemporal lobar degeneration. *Hum Mol Genet* 15(20), 2988–3001.

Geldmacher DS, Whitehouse PJ Jr (1997). Differential diagnosis of Alzheimer's disease. *Neurology* 48(suppl 6), S2–9.

Hosler BA, Siddique T, Sapp PC, et al (2000). Linkage of familial amyotrophic lateral sclerosis with frontotemporal dementia to chromosome 9q21-q22. *JAMA* 284(13), 1664–9.

Hsiung GYR, Sadovnick AD (2007). Genetics and dementia: risk factors, diagnosis and management. *Alzheimers Dement* 3, 418–27.

Huff FJ, Auerbach J, Chakravarti A, Boller F (1988). Risk of dementia in relatives of patients with Alzheimer's disease. *Neurology* 38, 786–90.

Hutton M, Lendon CL, Rizzu P, et al (1998). Association of missense and 5'-splice-site mutations in tau with the inherited dementia FTDP-17. *Nature* 393(6686), 702–5.

Jarvik L, LaRue A, Blacker D, et al (2008). Children of persons with Alzheimer disease. What does the future hold? *Alzheimer Dis Assoc Disord* 22, 6–20.

Jayadev S, Steinbart EJ, Chi YY, Kukull WA, Schellenberg GD, Bird TD (2008). Conjugal Alzheimer disease. *Arch Neurol* 65, 373–8.

Korten AE, Jorm AF, Henderson AS, Broe GA, Creasey H, McCusker E (1993). Assessing the risk of Alzheimer's disease in first-degree relatives of Alzheimer's disease cases. *Psychol Med* 23, 915–23.

Kurz MW, Schlitter AM, Larsen JP, Ballard C, Aarsland D (2006). Familial occurrence of dementia and parkinsonism: a systematic review. [Review] *Dement Geriatr Cogn Disord* 22(4), 288–95.

Lawson K, Wiggins S, Green T, Adam S, Bloch M, Hayden MR (1996). Adverse psychological events occurring in the first year after predictive testing for Huntington's disease. *J Med Genet* 33, 856–62.

Lee JH, Cheng R, Schupf N, et al (2007). The association between genetic variants in SORL1 and Alzheimer disease in an urban, multiethnic, community-based cohort. *Arch Neurol* 64, 501–6.

Lennox A, Karlinsky H, Meschino W, Buchanan JA, Percy ME, Berg JM (1994). Molecular genetic predictive testing for Alzheimer's disease: deliberations and preliminary recommendations. *Alzheimer Dis Assoc Disord* 8, 126–47.

Li H, Wetten S, St-Jean PL, et al (2008). Candidate single-nucleotide polymorphisms from a genomewide association study of Alzheimer disease. *Arch Neurol* 65, doi: 10.1001/archneurol.2007.3.

Mackenzie IR, Baker M, Pickering-Brown S, et al (2006). The neuropathology of frontotemporal lobar degeneration caused by mutations in the progranulin gene. [see comment]. *Brain* 129(pt 11), 3081–90.

Mayeux R, Saunders AM, Shea S, et al (1998). Utility of the apolipoprotein E genotype in the diagnosis of Alzheimer's disease. *N Engl J Med* 338, 506–11.

Medical and Scientific Committee ADI, Brodaty H, Conneally M, et al (1996). Consensus statement on predictive testing. *Alzheimer Dis Assoc Disord* 9, 182–7.

Meyer MR, Tschanz JT, Norton MC, et al (1998). APOE genotype predicts when – not whether – one is predisposed to develop Alzheimer disease. *Nature Genet* 19, 321–2.

Owen M, Liddell M, McGuffin P (1994). Alzheimer's disease. *BMJ* 308, 672–3.

Poirier J, Delisle MC, Quirion R, et al (1995). Apolipoprotein E4 allele as a predictor of cholinergic deficits and treatment outcome in Alzheimer disease. *Proc Natl Acad Sci U S A* 92, 12260–4.

Poirier J, Gauthier S (2008). Pharmacogenomics and the treatment of sporadic Alzheimer's disease. *Curr Pharmacogenom Personal Med* 6, 63–78.

Relkin NR, Tanzi R, Breitner J, et al (1996). Apolipoprotein E genotyping in Alzheimer's disease. *Lancet* 347, 1091–5.

Rogaeva E, Meng Y, Lee JH, et al (2007). The neuronal sortilin-related receptor SORL I is genetically associated with Alzheimer disease. *Nat Genet* 39, 168–77.

Roses AD (1996). Apolipoprotein E alleles as risk factors in Alzheimer's disease. *Annu Rev Med* 47, 387–400.

Roses AD (1997). Genetic testing for Alzheimer disease. Practical and ethical issues. *Arch Neurol* 54(10), 1226–9.

Rosso SM, Donker Kaat L, Baks T, et al (2003). Frontotemporal dementia in The Netherlands: patient characteristics and prevalence estimates from a population-based study. *Brain* 126(pt 9), 2016–22.

Rossor MN, Fox NC, Beck J, Campbell TC, Collinge J (1996). Incomplete penetrance of familial Alzheimer's disease in a pedigree with a novel presenilin-1 gene mutation. *Lancet* 347, 1560.

Scourfield J, Soldan J, Gray J, Houlihan G, Harper PS (1997). Huntington's disease: psychiatric practice in molecular genetic prediction and diagnosis. *Br J Psychiatry* 170, 146–9.

Seshadri S, Drachman DA, Lippa CF (1995). Apolipoprotein E B44 allele and the lifetime risk of Alzheimer's disease — What physicians know, and what they should know. *Arch Neurol* 52, 1074–9.

Singleton AB, Wharton A, O'Brien KK, et al (2002). Clinical and neuropathological correlates of apolipoprotein E genotype in dementia with Lewy bodies. [Comparative Study] *Dement Geriatr Cogn Disord* 14(4), 167–75.

Snowden JS, Neary D, Mann DMA (1996) *Fronto-Temporal Lobar Degeneration: Fronto-Temporal Dementia, Progressive Aphasia, Semantic Dementia*. Edinburgh, UK: Churchill Livingstone; 1–227.

Waring SC, Rosenberg RN (2008). Genome-wide association studies in Alzheimer's disease. *Arch Neurol* 65, 329–34.

Welsh-Bohmer KA, Gearing M, Saunders AM, Roses AD, Mirra S (1997). Apolipoprotein E genotypes in a neuropathological series from the consortium to establish a registry for Alzheimer's disease. *Ann Neurol* 42, 319–25.

Biomarkers

'Doctor, is there a blood test for Alzheimer's disease?'

This question is often asked by individuals with or without symptoms and by their relatives. The short answer is no, at this time, despite the advances made in the understanding of Alzheimer's disease (AD) and the insights yielded by molecular biology which may, in the not-too-distant future, result in specific disease-modifying treatments (see chapter 7). There are, however, other possible clinical implications that result from a greater understanding of pathogenesis. Most important of these is the possibility that this work will contribute to some form of molecular test. In chapter 1, we discussed the difficulties of clinical diagnosis and the importance of making an accurate assessment of disease type and severity. With the advent of specific therapies for AD, it is now incumbent upon clinicians to diagnose AD in the very early stages, to distinguish between the different causes of dementia, and to monitor the course of the condition. This would be much easier if a test were available that would identify patients early – perhaps even before a dementia was clinically apparent. A useful test would be one that allowed the clinician to monitor the progression of the disease accurately and without bias, or that could distinguish between AD and other dementias.

A test 'for' AD could predict onset of AD, assess severity of AD, or simply test for the presence of AD. While no test has been identified that fulfils any of these criteria yet, there are some promising developments from the fields of molecular biology and from neuroimaging which will be summarised in this chapter, an update of chapter 5 written by Simon Lovestone in the first edition of this book. This is a fast evolving topic and an excellent review of the field is that of Hampel et al, 2008.

Molecular biomarkers

There is great interest in finding a specific and sensitive molecular biomarker for AD. Ideally, the level of this marker would change over time and may therefore provide a marker of the start or perhaps the progression of disease. A series of proteins that might be relevant to AD have been examined in both blood and in cerebrospinal fluid (CSF). While none have at present a proven clinical use, the results so far have been encouraging to researchers in the area and it is possible that a molecular test will result. The undisputed facts for now are that AD, even in very early stage, is associated with lower β-amyloid peptide Aβ42 and higher *tau* levels in CSF (Galasko, 2007). The strength of this evidence is such that CSF examination has been proposed in the revised National Institute of Neurological and Communicative Disorders and Stroke-Alzheimer's Disease and Related Disorders Association

(NINCDS-ADRDA) criteria for AD as one of the tests to be considered (Dubois et al, 2007).

Tau is a normal microtubule-associated protein that is deposited, in a highly phosphorylated state, in the tangles that were recognised as critical to the pathology of the condition by Dr Alzheimer. Unfortunately, for the prospects of *tau* as a molecular biomarker test, *tau* is expressed in neurons only and so can only be accessed in CSF. In probably the best study, a formula based upon Aβ42, total tau and phosphorylated tau was highly predictive of the development of AD in a large prospectively followed cohort of patients with mild cognitive impairment (Hansson et al, 2006), suggesting that a combination of amyloid and tau measures may give the most accurate results. Other potentially promising CSF biomarkers include APP-cleaving enzyme (BACE) (Verheijen et al, 2006) and isoprostane (Irizarry et al, 2007). Amyloid and tau levels also appear to be similarly altered in the CSF of patients with dementia with Lewy bodies (Mollenahuer et al, 2006) and preliminary data indicated that α-synuclein can be measured and is significantly lowered in these individuals (Aarsland et al, 2008).

Amyloid, in contrast to *tau*, is ubiquitously expressed. Products of the amyloid precursor gene can thus be measured in blood as well as in CSF and could also reflect the start of the disease, although there are still doubts as to the sensitivity of the measurement of amyloid by-products in plasma (Graff-Radford et al, 2007; Sundelöf et al, 2008). Another avenue being explored is signaling proteins in plasma, related to hematopoiesis, immune response, apoptosis and neural support (Ray et al, 2008). Similarly, panels of candidate biomarkers are being studied in CSF using proteomic profiling (Simonsen et al, 2007).

Neuroimaging as a biomarker

Structural neuroimaging is routine in the diagnostic work-up for patients with dementia (Bastos et al, 2007). Most often CT or MRI is used to exclude other causes of cognitive impairment – tumors and strokes for example. For a diagnosis of AD, neuroimaging is not required by all (but it is by most) diagnostic guidelines, whereas for vascular dementia it is clearly part of the diagnostic process. In research, structural neuroimaging has proved invaluable and a number of attempts have been made to quantify and formally assess the atrophic changes seen. In general, these methods have little application in diagnosis. However, a number of interesting developments take neuroimaging beyond research and beyond simply supporting diagnosis and excluding treatable causes.

Structural imaging – CT and MRI

One of the promising developments in neuroimaging was specific imaging of the medial temporal lobe using axial CT scans (20–25B0 anterior to the normal angle). This angle allows quantification of medial temporal lobe atrophy – one of the earliest sites of AD pathology – and both cross-sectional and longitudinal studies were encouraging in finding a more than 90% accuracy rate (Nagy et al, 1999). Unfortunately, a study suggested that although differentiating dementia from normality, the method does not help in differential diagnosis (O'Brien et al, 2000) as a proportion of even normal elderly individuals has hippocampal atrophy (e.g. 30% of all elderly and nearly half of all very elderly in one study) (De Leon et al, 1997). Similarly, whilst most studies report that hippocampal atrophy can be used to differentiate AD from vascular dementia (Libon et al, 1998; O'Brien et al, 1997), others found that rates of atrophy of cortical structures are similar in the two conditions (Pantel et al, 1998).

MRI has a number of distinct advantages over CT – in particular in the improved resolution and the visualisation of soft tissues. MRI is without question the method of choice for imaging white matter pathology. Just as in CT, the atrophy of AD is readily detectable by MRI but less readily differentiated from normal ageing. Even so correct identification of AD patients relative to normals is 88% (O'Brien, 1995), better than the 80% to 85% of CT but at considerably increased scanning time and expense. These medial lobe changes take place early in the disease process and may therefore be a good biomarker for early change (Bobinski et al, 1999). In line with these findings, many studies have assessed whether

MRI will help to predict which individuals with mild cognitive impairment are likely to convert to full dementia. In a longitudinal study, a number of MRI measures, in particular atrophy of the entorhinal cortex and the caudal part of the anterior cingulate, were found to differ between individuals who over a 3-year period remained mildly impaired but within the normal range and those who converted to either full dementia or questionable dementia (Killiany et al, 2000). Discriminant function analyses showed greatest separation between normals and converters (accuracy of 93%) than between questionables and converters (75%). Other studies also indicated that MRI visualisation of the medial temporal lobe might be a useful means both to identify those at high genetic risk of developing dementia and those with mild cognitive impairment of converting to dementia.

Quantification of atrophy using MRI can be performed using a variety of approaches but one of the most promising is that of serial registration – the comparison of scans, mathematically and visually, taken some time apart. Fox et al have used this approach to show that the rate of brain atrophy in a group with AD was 2.37% per year, while in normal controls it was 0.41% per year (Fox et al, 2000). Usefully, they translated these figures into power calculations assuming that serial registration was to be used as a biomarker of disease progression. If this is done based on their figures, then 200 patients would have to be recruited into each arm of a placebo-controlled trial to have 90% power to detect a drug effect equivalent to a 20% reduction in the rate of atrophy. Such numbers are achievable and serial registration may prove to be a useful biomarker in such trials. This has high relevance to trials using potentially disease-modifying drugs (see chapter 7).

MRI certainly has a role to play in differential diagnosis but it is no more definitive than CT. Thus no differences were found between dementia with Lewy bodies (DLB) and AD (Barber et al, 2000) and even in frontotemporal dementia (FTD), where there are clear volumetric differences at post-mortem. It is, however, the relevance of vascular changes in general and white matter changes in particular that is most problematical. Periventricular lucency and white matter hyperintensities are common in the elderly, and also in depression (Barber et al, 1999). These white matter lesions are more common in groups of elderly with dementia but that is not of much help when faced with an individual patient. Their relevance to diagnosis or to measure change remains to be fully established.

Biochemical imaging – magnetic resonance spectroscopy

Magnetic resonance spectroscopy (MRS) is an imaging modality that can be used to measure biochemical change in the living brain, including the neuronal marker N-acetyl aspartate (NAA) (Koller et al, 1984); creatine, which is involved in phosphate metabolism; choline containing substances (e.g. phosphocholine and glycerophosphocholine), which are crucial to membrane metabolism; and *myo*-inositol, which significantly affects neuronal survival. MRS has been shown, for example, to detect elevations in myo-inositol occurring before dementia in individuals with AD (Huang et al, 1999) and along with creatinine and NAA to correlate with cognition in late-onset AD (Rose et al, 1999). Some evidence suggests altered ^{1}H MRS markers in AD and studies of AD populations have reported reductions in NAA, which is correlated with disease severity, and increases in choline and *myo*-inositol (Schuff et al, 1998). Moreover, reduced levels of NAA and increased levels of *myo*-inositol characterised AD with 83% sensitivity and 98% specificity. On the other hand, MRS has not panned out to be a major tool in AD research, contrary to PET.

Functional imaging – SPECT and PET

Single photon emission computerized tomography (SPECT) can be used to measure blood flow and receptor density amongst other outputs. The method requires injection of a radiotracer, although the amount of radiation emitted is low. SPECT has been used to show parietal and temporal pattern of loss in AD

(Wyper et al, 1993) but it is really in the differential diagnosis of AD and FTD that SPECT becomes invaluable. Differentiating between the two can be difficult and the SPECT scan is the investigation of choice to detect the profound frontal blood flow loss that occurs early in the condition (Charpentier et al, 2000). Future studies using SPECT to image particular functional subsets of neurons will be of interest (Nobuhara et al, 2000).

Positron emission tomography (PET) has become more available than expected a decade ago, and the availability of ligands that may be specific to amyloid has increased its relevance to early diagnosis (Nordberg, 2007). The initial observations using PET in AD were altered blood flow, altered glucose metabolism and altered receptor density (Blin et al, 1993; Guze et al, 1991; Kumar et al, 1991). These changes are present very early on in the course of disease and a seminal study showed that those at mild genetic risk of AD had abnormal PET scans decades before the age of onset (Small et al, 1996). More recent work has clarified the potential value of fluorodeoxyglucose (FDG) PET as an early diagnostic marker (Jagust et al, 2007), sufficiently so that it is one of the tests under validation for the revised NINCDS-ADRDA criteria for AD (Dubois et al, 2007). It remains to be established if the amyloid ligands such as the Pittsburg Compound B (PIB; Klunk et al, 2004) and others under development will have sufficient specificity and sensitivity to be used as early diagnostic markers of AD, and possibly markers of response to treatment using amyloid-modifying drugs.

Conclusion

At present, there is no blood test for AD. CSF biomarkers are promising but lumbar puncture remains a relatively invasive procedure to study Aβ protein fragments and *tau*. Structural neuroimaging is useful to exclude certain unusual causes of dementia where these may be suspected following an examination. Structural neuroimaging can be helpful in differential diagnosis although the changes – atrophy and white matter changes are also common in the elderly. Functional imaging is particularly helpful in differentiating FTD from AD. Promising advances include those that systematically compare serial scans and those that quantify or image the medial temporal lobe. The findings that there are MRI and PET changes decades before the disease do confirm the findings in mild cognitive impairment that imaging may well be useful as a marker of disease change and of prediction of conversion to dementia.

Summary

- Biomarkers for the presence of disease or for monitoring the progression of the disease are eagerly awaited but not yet available.
- Structural imaging by CT or MRI can be used to aid differential diagnosis.

- Structural imaging of the medial temporal lobe may be useful in predicting conversion to dementia.
- Serial MRI scans may be useful in monitoring change.
- Functional imaging, especially SPECT, is helpful in diagnosis of frontal lobe dementia.
- Functional imaging using FDG and PET can allow for an earlier diagnosis of AD in symptomatic individuals.

References

Aarsland D, Kurz M, Beyer M, Bronnick K, Piepenstock Nore S, Ballard C (2008). Early discriminatory diagnosis of dementia with Lewy bodies. The emerging role of CSF and imaging biomarkers. *Dement Geriatr Cogn Disord* 25, 195–205.

Barber R, Ballard C, McKeith IG, Gholkar A, O'Brien J (2000). MRI volumetric study of dementia with Lewy bodies – A comparison with AD and vascular dementia. *Neurology* 54, 1304–9.

Barber R, Scheltens F, Gholkar A, et al (1999). White matter lesions on magnetic resonance imaging in dementia with Lewy bodies, Alzheimer's disease, vascular dementia, and normal aging. *J Neurol Neurosurg Psychiatry* 67, 66–72.

Bastos Leite AJ, Barkhof F, Scheltens P (2007). Structural brain imaging. In: Gauthier S, ed. *Clinical Diagnosis and Management of Alzheimer's Disease*, 3rd edn. Abingdon, UK, Informa Healthcare; 81–96.

Blin J, Baron JC, Dubois B, et al (1993). Loss of brain 5-HT2 receptors in Alzheimer's disease. *Brain* 116, 497–510.

Bobinski M, De Leon MJ, Convit A, et al (1999). MRI of entorhinal cortex in mild Alzheimer's disease. *Lancet* 353, 38–40.

Charpentier P, Lavenu I, Defebvre L, et al (2000). Alzheimer's disease and frontotemporal dementia are differentiated by discriminant analysis applied to 99 mTc HmPAO SPECT data. *J Neurol Neurosurg Psychiatry* 69, 661–3.

De Leon MJ, George AE, Golomb J, et al (1997). Frequency of hippocampal formation atrophy in normal aging and Alzheimer's disease. *Neurobiol Aging* 18, 1–11.

Dubois B, Feldman HH, Jacova C, et al (2007). Research criteria for the diagnosis of Alzheimer's disease: revising the NINCDS-ADRDA criteria. *Lancet Neurol* 6, 734–46.

Fox NC, Cousens S, Scahill R, Harvey RJ, Rossor MN (2000). Using serial registered brain magnetic resonance imaging to measure disease progression in Alzheimer disease: power calculations and estimates of sample size to detect treatment effects. *Arch Neurol* 57, 339–44.

Galasko D (2007). Biological markers. In: Gauthier S, ed. *Clinical Diagnosis and Management of Alzheimer's Disease*, 3rd edn. Abingdon, UK, Informa Healthcare; 125–133.

Graff-Radford NR, Crook JE, Lucas J, et al (2007). Association of low plasma Aß42/ Aß40 ratios with increased imminent risk for mild cognitive impairment and Alzheimer disease. *Arch Neurol* 64, 354–62.

Guze BH, Baxter LRJ, Schwartz JM, Szuba MP, Mazziotta JC, Phelps ME (1991). Changes in glucose metabolism in dementia of the Alzheimer type compared with depression: a preliminary report. *Psychiatry Res* 40, 195–202.

Hampel H, Bürger K, Teipel SJ, Bokde ALW, Zetterberg H, Blennow K (2008). Core candidate neurochemical and imaging biomarkers of Alzheimer's disease. *Alzheimers Dement* 4, 38–48.

Hansson O, Zetterberg H, Buchhave P, Londos F, Blennow K, Minthon L (2006). Association between CSF biomarkers and incipient Alzheimer's disease in patients with mild cognitive impairment: a follow-up study. *Lancet Neurol* 5, 228–34.

Huang W, Alexander GE, Daly EM, et al (1999). High brain myo-inositol levels in the predementia phase of Alzheimer's disease in adults with Down's syndrome: A 1 H MRS study. *Am J Psychiatry* 156, 1879–86.

Irizarry MC, Yao Y, Hyman BT, Growdon JH, Pratico D (2007). Plasma F2 A isoprostane levels in Alzheimer's and Parkinson's disease. *Neurodegener Dis* 4, 403–5.

Jagust W, Reed B, Mungas D, Ellis W, DeCarli C (2007). What does fluorodeoxyglucose PET imaging add to a clinical diagnosis of dementia? *Neurology* 69, 871–7.

Killiany RJ, Gomez-Isla T, Moss M, et al (2000). Use of structural magnetic resonance imaging to predict who will get Alzheimer's disease. *Ann Neurol* 47, 430–9.

Klunk WE, Engler H, Nordberg A, et al (2004). Imaging brain amyloid in Alzheimer's disease with Pittsburg Compound-B. *Ann Neurol* 55, 306–19.

Koller KJ, Zaczek R, Coyle JT (1984). N-acetyl-aspartyl-glutamate: regional levels in rat brain and the effects of brain lesions as determined by a new HPLC method. *J Neurochem* 43, 1136–42.

Kumar A, Schapiro MB, Grady C, et al (1991). High-resolution PET studies in Alzheimer's disease. *Neuropsychopharmacology* 4, 35–46.

Libon DJ, Bogdanoff B, Cloud BS, et al (1998). Declarative and procedural learning, quantitative measures of the hippocampus, and subcortical white alterations in Alzheimer's disease and ischaemic vascular dementia. *J Clin Exp Neuropsychol* 20, 30–41.

Mollenhauer B, Trenkwalder C, von Ahsen N, et al (2006) Beta-amlyoid 1–42 and tau-protein in cerebrospinal fluid of patients with Parkinson's disease dementia. *Dement Geriatr Cogn Disord* 22, 200–8.

Nagy Z, Hindley NJ, Braak H, et al (1999). Relationship between clinical and radiological diagnostic criteria for Alzheimer's disease and the extent of neuropathology as reflected by 'stages': a prospective study. *Dement Geriatr Cogn Disord* 10, 109–14.

Nobuhara K, Halldin C, Hall H, et al (2000). Z-IQNP: a potential radioligand for SPECT imaging of muscarinic acetylcholine receptors in Alzheimer's disease. *Psychopharmacology (Berl)* 149, 45–55.

Nordberg A (2007). Functional brain imaging. In: Gauthier S, ed. *Clinical Diagnosis and Management of Alzheimer's Disease*, 3rd edn. Informa Healthcare; 97–110.

O'Brien JT (1995). Is hippocampal atrophy on magnetic resonance imaging a marker for Alzheimer's disease? *Int J Geriatr Psychiatry* 10, 431–5.

O'Brien JT, Desmond P, Ames D, Schweitzer I, Chiu E, Tress B (1997). Temporal lobe magnetic resonance Imaging can differentiate Alzheimer's disease from normal ageing, depression, vascular dementia and other causes of cognitive impairment. *Psychol Med* 27, 1267–75.

O'Brien JT, Metcalfe S, Swann A, et al (2000). Medial temporal lobe width on CT scanning in Alzheimer's disease: comparison with vascular dementia, depression and dementia with Lewy bodies. *Dement Geriatr Cogn Disord* 11, 114–8.

Pantel J, Schröder J, Essig M, et al (1998). In vivo quantification of brain volumes in subcortical vascular dementia and Alzheimer's disease – An MRI-based study. *Dementia* 9, 309–16.

Ray S, Britschgi M, Herbert C, et al (2008). Classification and prediction of clinical Alzheimer's diagnosis based on plasma signaling protein. Nature Medicine published on line 14 Oct 2007; doi: 10.1038/nm1653.

Rose SE, De Zubicaray GI, Wang DM, et al (1999). A 1 H MRS study of probable Alzheimer's disease and normal aging: implications for longitudinal monitoring of dementia progression. *Magn Reson Imaging* 17, 291–19.

Schuff N, Amend DL, Meyerhoff DJ, et al (1998). Alzheimer disease: quantitative H-1 MR spectroscopic imaging of frontoparietal brain. *Radiology* 207, 91–102.

Simonsen AH, Mcguire J, Hansson O, et al (2007). Novel panel of cerebrospinal fluid biomarkers for the prediction of progression to Alzheimer dementia in patients with mild cognitive impairment. *Arch Neurol* 64, 366–70.

Small GW, Komo S, La Rue A, et al (1996). Early detection of Alzheimer's disease by combining apolipoprotein E and neuroimaging. *Ann N Y Acad Sci* 802, 70–8.

Sundelöf J, Giedraitis MC, Irizarry MC, et al (2008). Plasma ß amyloid and the risk of Alzheimer disease and dementia in elderly men. *Arch Neurol* 65, 256–63.

Verheijen JH, Huisman LG, van Lent N,et al (2006). Detection of a soluble form of BACE-1 in human cerebrospinal fluid by a sensitive activity assay. *Clin Chem* 52, 1168–74

Wyper D, Teasdale E, Patterson J, et al (1993). Abnormalities in rCBF and computed tomography in patients with Alzheimer's disease and in controls. *Br J Radiol* 66, 23–7.

Symptomatic treatments for dementia

'Doctor, do you have a treatment to help my mother's memory?'

The current chapter discusses symptomatic treatments for dementia. The predominant focus is the licensed pharmaceutical treatments for Alzheimer's disease (AD), but key issues are also outlined for non-AD dementias, other symptomatic treatments for which there is clinical trial evidence, natural remedies and non-pharmacological treatments. The boundary between symptomatic treatments and potentially disease-modifying remedies is blurred, as it depends both upon the proposed mechanism of action and the type of evidence available from clinical trials. For example, there are no broadly accepted surrogate measures for tracking disease modification over the longitudinal course of AD, although increasing evidence highlights the potential utility of neuroimaging and cerebrospinal fluid (CSF) biomarkers. In addition, there is an ongoing debate about the type and length of sustained benefit which is necessary to suggest disease modification rather than just symptomatic benefit. The selection of 'symptomatic therapies' in the current chapter is therefore based on personal judgement. The agents discussed are limited to those where there has been at least some evidence of potential benefit and focuses predominantly on cholinesterase inhibitors and memantine, with brief discussion of other cholinergic therapies and non-pharmacological approaches (Table 6.1). These are included as there are no postulated mechanisms specific to the AD process, although as highlighted in the discussion of cholinesterase inhibitors, these issues are far from clear even for drug therapies which most people would consider to be 'symptomatic'.

Symptomatic pharmaceutical treatments for AD

There are two classes of drug approved for the treatment of AD. The cholinesterase inhibitors tacrine, donepezil, rivastigmine and galantamine are licensed for the treatment of mild-to-moderate AD and the NMDA receptor antagonist memantine is licensed for the treatment of moderate-to-severe AD. In some countries donepezil is also approved for severe AD, based on Winblad et al, 2006 study.

Cholinesterase inhibitors

There is evidence from more than 30 randomised clinical trials of cholinesterase inhibitors in various stages of AD with a variety of different outcome measures (e.g. Rogers et al, 1998; Rösler et al, 1999. In systematic meta-analyses (Birks et al, 2007; Loy and Schneider 2007; Birks and Harvey 2007), each of the three widely prescribed cholinesterase inhibitors (donepezil, rivastigmine, galanthamine) conferred significant benefit compared to placebo for the treatment of mild-to-moderate AD in the treatment of cognitive deficits (Alzheimer's disease assessment scale—cognitive subscale [ADAS-COG] advantages compared to placebo: 1.3–4.4 points). Because of the wide number of different methods and scales used, it is more difficult to quantify the improvements in activities of daily living and global outcome across trials, but they are highly significant for all three drugs. Of note, the mean level of cognitive performance remains above baseline for 6 to 12 months in most studies. A more recent trial examining a different formulation of rivastigmine, the transdermal patch, demonstrated a similar level of efficacy in a large placebo-controlled trial (Winblad et al, 2007).

Although only a handful of studies have maintained a placebo-controlled design for more than 6 months, the initial evidence is encouraging with placebo-controlled trials showing continued benefit over 12 (Winblad et al, 2001) and 24 months (Courtney et al, 2004). The majority of trials have focused upon people with mild-to-moderate AD, although work examining the value of cholinesterase therapy in people with more severe AD indicated significant cognitive and functional benefits associated with treatment

Table 6.1
Level of Evidence for Different Therapies from Randomised, Placebo-Controlled Trials

	MCI	AD	DLB/PDD	VaD
Cholinesterase inhibitors	−	+++	+++	++
Memantine	−	+++	+	++
Vitamin E[a]	−	+	−	−
Gingko Biloba[a]	−	+	−	−
Cognitive stimulation and related therapies	+	+++	−	−

[a] Vitamin E and Gingko Biloba are discussed in chapter 7.
Abbreviations: − no evidence, + marginal evidence, ++ some evidence but insufficient to recommend for clinical practice, + + + robust evidence from clinical trials.

(Feldman et al, 2001; Windlad et al, 2006; Howard et al, 2007). However, the trials conducted so far do not indicate that in general cholinesterase inhibitors significantly delay the onset of dementia in people with mild cognitive impairment (MCI), although further work is needed to determine whether there is benefit in MCI patients carrying the apolipoprotein E4 (Petersen et al, 2005) or the butyrylcholinesterase K (Feldman et al, 2007) genotypes.

Cholinesterase inhibitors are safe and generally well tolerated in AD provided sensible exclusions are made, such as patients with symptomatic bradycardia. Gastrointestinal side effects are the most frequent, with nausea occurring in 10% to 30% of people, sometimes associated with vomiting. For the majority of individuals, the effects are transient or giving the medication with food is sufficient to resolve or improve

the symptoms. Sometimes, it is necessary to use a lower dose or change between individual cholinesterase inhibitors, as tolerance to different drugs may vary for individual patients. It is rare in our experience for it to be necessary to discontinue treatment because of adverse events. There has been some concern about the possibility of a slightly increased mortality risk in people with MCI treated with cholinesterase inhibitors (Mayor 2005), which is another important reason to be restrained about the use of cholinesterase inhibitors in these individuals. There is no increased mortality risk in relation to cholinesterase inhibitors for people with AD.

There has been considerable debate about whether the magnitude of the symptomatic improvements is substantial enough to impact meaningfully on quality of life. The absence of formal quality-of-life measures in the majority of clinical trials is disappointing and does make it difficult to address this issue. A survey completed by the Alzheimer's Society in the United Kingdom, which included more than 2000 carers of people with AD taking anti-dementia drugs, highlighted that the majority of people feel that the treatments did give them meaningful improvements (Ballard et al, 2007a). More systematic evidence comes from Goal Attainment Scaling, which enables people to choose the outcome measures most important to them as the primary evaluation for clinical trials. Using this approach, Rockwood and colleagues demonstrated in a placebo-controlled trial of the cholinesterase inhibitor galantamine that key goals were significantly more likely to be achieved amongst people taking galantamine compared to the placebo-treated individuals (Rockwood et al, 2006).

Who to treat, for how long and which drug?

A number of trials, mostly open label and of short duration, have failed to demonstrate any consistent pattern of differences in the efficacy between individual drugs (e.g. Wilcock et al, 2003; Wilkinson et al, 2003; Jones et al, 2003). Despite the suggestion from the Bullock et al study that patients with the butyrylcholinesterase wild type genotype may respond preferentially to rivastigmine this a largely a research question, but highlights that in the near future pharmacogenetics may enable us to direct therapy more effectively.

There is evidence of more severe gastrointestinal side effects with rivastigmine than the other agents, particularly in studies with rapid titration, although the tolerability profile of rivastigmine is substantially better with the transdermal patch formulation (Winblad et al, 2007).

The evidence suggests that depending upon the audit criteria, 40% to 75% of patients experience a significant benefit from cholinesterase inhibitor therapy, but that it is extremely difficult to predict 'responders' in advance. The most pragmatic approach is therefore to offer all patients with mild-to-moderate AD a 6-month trial of treatment, unless there are clinical factors such as symptomatic bradycardia or serious concerns about safe administration of the medication. Defining response is difficult, since for individual patients the course of the disease without treatment is unknown. Most treatment guidelines emphasise stability or improvement in cognition and/or function and clinical judgement of stabilisation are made by the discussion with the people and their family, although more innovative approaches such as a simplified form of goal attainment scaling have also been used. Determining whether there is continuing benefits from longer term therapy is even more difficult given the greater uncertainties about clinical outcome without therapy. Some authorities have advocated a trial discontinuation of treatment as a method of determining whether there is ongoing treatment response. This approach is not based on any robust evidence, and it can be very difficult to distinguish loss of benefit from withdrawal effects which can include marked exacerbation of behavioural symptoms (Holmes et al, 2004). Our view is that these guidelines in general are over-complicating the situation, and it is essentially a clinical judgement.

Views differ about whether individuals who do not respond to an adequate treatment trial or who are unable to tolerate the medication should be discontinued or changed to an alternative therapy. When tolerability is the main issue, clinical experience certainly suggests that another drug from the same class may be better tolerated. The evidence for 'switching' between different cholinesterase inhibitors for lack of efficacy is limited and based upon open or retrospective studies (e.g. Bullock and Connolly, 2002; Wilkinson and Howe, 2005). There is one case report of a fatal adverse event during transition from donepezil to rivastigmine (Taylor et al, 2002). In clinical practice, other people may increase the dose of a cholinesterase inhibitor above the British national formulary (BNF) recommended dose limits, but there is a very limited information regarding the safety or efficacy of this approach. The other potential approach of combination therapy with a cholinesterase inhibitor and memantine is discussed in the section of the chapter pertaining to memantine.

Other cholinergic therapies

Several muscarinic agonists have been evaluated in clinical trials, with some evidence of efficacy, but poor gastrointestinal and cardiovascular tolerability (e.g. Bodick et al, 1997). Other muscarinic agonists are in development, but none are licensed for the clinical treatment of AD. Nicotine confers short-term improvements in attention (Sahakian et al, 1989), and the allosteric modulation of nicotinic receptors by galantamine has been suggested as part of its mode of action (Maelicke 2000). Other nicotinic agents are currently being evaluated in clinical trials.

Disease modification

Recent work has considered the key issue of whether cholinesterase inhibitors or other cholinergic therapies may also have a disease-modifying impact, and in particular whether they impact upon β-amyloid (Aβ) deposits in the cortex. There are several strong pieces of evidence from experimental studies showing that cholinesterase inhibitors and other cholinergic therapies reduce the accumulation of amyloid in cultured neurones and in rodent models (e.g. Gu et al, 2003; Verhoeff 2005). More recently, there is exciting new evidence from small clinical trials using CSF biomarkers supporting the conclusions of the experimental work. For example, Aβ concentrations in CSF from patients were reduced twofold after administration of the muscarinic M1 receptor agonist talsaclidine for four weeks in a double-blind, placebo-controlled trial of 40 patients (Hock et al, 2003). In a further pilot clinical study comparing 27 cholinesterase inhibitor–treated AD patients with matched untreated patients for one year, increases in CSF Aβ were prevented by both rivatigamine and tacrine treatment (Darreh-Shori et al, 2002). In the first human autopsy study examining the impact of cholinesterase inhibitor therapy upon amyloid pathology in the brain, 12 dementia with Lewy body (DLB) patients treated with cholinesterase inhibitors as part of placebo-controlled trials were compared to 12 matched untreated patients, demonstrating that DLB patients treated with cholinesterase inhibitors had 68% less parenchymal Aβ deposition in the cerebral cortex than untreated patients, a statistically significant difference (Ballard et al, 2007a). Consistent with these data, a recent clinical trial demonstrated a reduction in the progression of hippocampal atrophy on MRI in cholinesterase inhibitor–treated AD patients (Hashimoto M et al, 2005). Further work is needed, but there is increasing evidence that cholinesterase inhibitors may have an impact upon disease pathology.

Memantine

NMDA receptors

In addition to loss of function of particular subsets, one theory that has attracted attention for many years in AD and other neurodegenerative conditions is the possibility that over-activity of excitatory amino acid transmitters may be related to neurotoxicity that occurs in these conditions. While there is loss of glutamatergic pyramidal neurons, there is no loss of glutamate binding sites – in particular NMDA receptor sites (Cowburn et al, 1990). This led to the hypothesis that a slow over-stimulation of NMDA and non-NMDA glutamate receptors may contribute to loss of neurons in AD and that this may precede the formation of amyloid plaques and other aspects of pathology (Beal, 1992). An alternative view was that neurons would be rendered more vulnerable to excitotoxic damage if exposed to amyloid, and this view was certainly substantiated by experiments with cells in culture (Gray and Patel, 1995; Mattson et al, 1992). NMDA excitotoxicity also seems to have a relation with the other component of AD pathology, because treatment of neurons with glutamate increases tau phosphorylation at the same sites as in the AD brain (Couratier et al, 1996). Moreover, glutamate increases total tau expression levels (Esclaire et al, 1997). The effect of glutamate then is to increase the amount of free tau both through increasing expression and through increasing phosphorylation. It is plausible that this increase in free tau may increase tau aggregation into neurofibrillary tangles.

Because of the known neurotoxicity of excitatory amino acids, a number of NMDA inhibitors have been developed for use in chronic disorders like AD and also in acute disorders such as stroke. High-potency NMDA antagonists have unwanted psychomimetic effects but low-potency antagonists are, in general, well tolerated. One such compound is memantine, which was in fact one of the first compounds to be assessed in AD (Fleischhacker et al, 1986).

Memantine hydrochloride, licensed for the treatment of moderate-to-severe AD, is a voltage-dependent, moderate-affinity uncompetitive NMDA-receptor antagonist that mirrors the role of physiological magnesium. Memantine has been extensively used in clinical practice in Germany for many years (Förstl, 2000) and licensed much more recently in other countries. Three randomised, placebo-controlled trials have examined memantine treatment (20 mg/day) over 24 to 28 weeks in moderate-to-severe AD, two trials comparing memantine with placebo and one comparing memantine to placebo in people already receiving stable therapy with donepezil. The meta-analysis indicated a significant beneficial effect at six months on cognition (2.97 points on the 100-point SIB, 95% CI 1.68 to 4.26 and $P < 0.00001$), activities of daily living (1.27 points on the 54-point ADCS-ADLsev, 95% CI 0.44 to 2.09 and $P = 0.003$) and clinical impression of change (0.28 points on the 7-point

CIBIC-Plus, 95% CI 0.15 to 0.41 and $P < 0.0001$) (McShane et al, 2007). Of note, an individual item analysis suggested better maintenance of key skills including mobility and feeding in patients taking memantine (Doody et al, 2004). The Tariot et al (2004) study, one of the three included in the meta-analysis, explored the addition of memantine or placebo to patients stable on donepezil in severe AD and showed a better outcome in the memantine group than in the placebo group after 24 weeks for measures of cognition (Severe Impairment Battery [SIB]), function (Alzheimer's disease cooperative study—activities of daily living [ADCS-ADL]), and global measure of change (CIBIC-Plus), with good tolerability. The three trials focusing on mild-to-moderate AD show benefits, however, these are less convincing (McShane et al, 2007).

Memantine is generally well tolerated, with no side effects occurring at a higher rate than seen with placebo treatment in the Cochrane meta-analysis (McShane et al, 2007). Side effects described as common in the data sheet include headache, tiredness and confusion, whilst anxiety, increased libido, hypertension and embolic events are also listed.

Similarly to cholinesterase inhibitors there is also emerging evidence regarding the possible impact of memantine upon disease pathology. Consistent with the proposed role of NMDA receptors, a longitudinal clinical study indicates that memantine therapy may reduce phosphorylated tau in the CSF (Degerman Gunnarsson et al, 2007).

In clinical practice, memantine is used much less frequently than cholinesterase inhibitors despite excellent tolerability and clinical trial evidence to suggest that key skills that are important to maintain quality of life are better preserved in people taking memantine. Therefore, there is a good case to use memantine in people with more severe AD, particularly as there may also be benefits with respect to neuropsychiatric and behavioural symptoms (see chapter 2). Adding memantine is probably also the most evidence-based approach to try and maintain benefit in patients who are losing their clinical response to cholinesterase inhibitor therapy.

Non-pharmacological treatments

A number of different approaches, including reminiscence therapy, reality orientation and cognitive stimulation (Woods et al, 2008; Spector et al, 2003; Spector et al, 2008; Orrell et al, 2005), combining elements of cognitive training, promoting well-being and social interaction in a group setting have consistently demonstrated modest but significant improvements (approximately 1 point on the Mini Mental State Examination [MMSE] or 2 points on the ADAS COG) in a total of 13 trials with a total of more than 450

participants. These studies have focused predominately upon people with dementia of moderate severity, and the utility in people with less severe cognitive impairment has not been systematically evaluated. A further important question is whether 'brain training' without the additional elements confers benefit. This is an area where further work is urgently needed, but important preliminary work demonstrates that benefits can be achieved in people with MCI (Belleville et al, 2006), although it is not yet clear whether they generalise to overall function.

Dementia with Lewy bodies and Parkinson's disease dementia

The pharmacological management of DLB and PDD presents a major clinical challenge, with multiple pharmacological treatments often required for the management of a range of clinical symptoms including motor parkinsonism, cognitive failure, psychiatric symptoms and autonomic dysfunction. For the management of parkisonian symptoms, levodopa monotherapy is the preferred option in DLB with response rates of about 50% (Bonelli et al, 2004), following the usual principle of 'start low, go slow'. Other anti-parkinsonian medications including selegeline, amantadine, catechol-o-methyltransferase (COMT) inhibitors, anticholinergics and dopamine agonists should usually be avoided because of concerns about inducing confusion and psychosis.

Placebo-, randomised-controlled trials of the cholinesterase inhibitor rivastigmine have demonstrated significant benefits for cognition, activities of daily living, neuropsychiatric symptoms and global outcome in DLB (McKeith et al, 2000) and PDD (Emre et al, 2004), supported by case series, cross-over trials and open studies with other cholinesterase inhibitors (e.g. Shea et al, 1998; Kaufer et al, 1998, Reading et al, 2001; Grace et al, 2001; Aarsland et al, 2002), and one study reporting a rebound worsening of neuropsychiatric symptoms, when treatment was stopped abruptly (Minett et al, 2003). Taken overall, the effects of the three available anticholinesterase inhibitors appear similar, with doses in the same range as used in AD, although the best level of evidence from placebo-controlled trials is for rivastigmine. The response of neuropsychiatric symptoms to cholinesterase inhibitor therapy is particularly important in view of the risk of severe neuroleptic sensitivity reactions in DLB (McKeith et al, 1992; Ballard et al, 1998) and PDD (Aarsland et al, 2005) patients. General tolerability of cholinesterase inhibitors is similar to that seen in AD, and reassuringly parkinsonian signs do not generally worsen on treatment. Case reports of the use of memantine in DLB are still very limited and some, with some indication of symptomatic

benefits and some concerns regarding the potential to worsen delusions and hallucinations (e.g. Sabbagh et al, 2005). Placebo-controlled trials of memantine in DLB are ongoing.

Drugs for vascular dementia

There have been a number of well-conducted 6 month randomised-controlled trials of cholinesterase inhibitors in mild-to-moderate vascular dementia (VaD) (e.g. Black et al, 2003; Wilkinson et al, 2003; Erkinjuntti et al, 2002). In general, these trials have consistently demonstrated cognitive benefits, but benefits for activities of daily living and global outcome have been disappointing. Post hoc sub-analyses indicate that there may be benefit in people with mixed VaD/AD (Ballard et al, 2008; Erkinjuntti et al, 2002), but less evidence of significant benefits in pure VaD. One recent trial indicates significant benefits for some aspects of cognition with donepezil in patients with cognitive impairment related to the genetic cerebrovasuclar condition CADASIL (Dichgans et al, 2008), indicating the potential for response to cholinesterase inhibitors in severe microvascular disease.

Memantine has also been evaluated in VaD in two randomised-controlled trials of 6 months' duration (Orgogozo et al, 2002; Wilcock et al, 2002), again with significant cognitive improvement that did not translate to global clinical benefits. A post-hoc analysis suggested that there is a possibility that memantine may be more effective in people with microvascular disease.

Conclusion

There is robust evidence base demonstrating that cholinesterase inhibitors and memantine confer significant symptomatic benefits in people with AD, and emerging evidence suggesting the possibility of disease modification. Cholinesterase inhibitors also confer significant clinical benefit in DLB and PDD, but there is currently insufficient evidence to recommend the treatment of VaD or MCI with cholinesterase inhibitor therapy.

Summary

- Cholinesterase inhibitors and memantine have been established as symptomatic treatment of AD.
- The value of these drugs in VaD is not fully established.
- Cholinesterase inhibitors have been established as symptomatic drugs for DLB and PDD.
- There has been no demonstrable benefit in MCI.
- There is uncertainty as to the potential of these drugs to modify disease progression after the diagnosis of dementia.

- Non-pharmacological approaches may be useful in the treatment of AD.

References

Aarsland D, Ballard C, Larsen JP, McKeith I, O'Brien J, Perry R (2005). Neuroleptic sensitivity in Parkinson's disease and parkinsonian dementias. *J Clin Psychiatry* 66(5), 633–7.

Aarsland D, Laake K, Larsen JP, Janvin C (2002). Donepezil for cognitive impairment in Parkinson's disease: a randomised controlled study. *J Neurol Neurosurg Psychiatry* 72, 708–12.

Ballard C, Grace J, McKeith I, Holmes C (1998). Neuroleptic sensitivity in dementia with Lewy bodies and Alzheimer's disease. *Lancet* 351(9108), 1032–3.

Ballard C, Sauter M, Scheltens P, et al (2008). Efficacy, safety and tolerability of rivastigmine capsules in patients with probable vascular dementia: the VantagE study. *Current Medical Research and Opinion* 24(9), 2561–74.

Ballard C, Sorensen S, Sharp S (2007a). Pharmacological therapy for people with Alzheimer's disease: the balance of clinical effectiveness, ethical issues and social and healthcare costs. *J Alzheimers Dis* 12(1), 53–9.

Ballard CG, Chalmers KA, Todd C, et al (2007b). Cholinesterase inhibitors reduce cortical Abeta in dementia with Lewy bodies. *Neurology* 68(20), 1726–9.

Beal MF (1992). Mechanisms of excitotoxicity in neurologic diseases. *FASEB J* 6, 3338–44.

Belleville S, Gilbert B, Fontaine F, Gagnon L, Menard E, Gauthier S (2006). Improvement of episodic memory in persons with mild cognitive impairment and healthy older adults: evidence from a cognitive intervention program. *Dement Geriatr Cogn Disord* 22(5–6), 486–99.

Birks J, Grimley Evans J, Iakovidou V, et al (2007). Rivastigmine for Alzheimer's disease. Cochrane Dementia and Cognitive Improvement Group. *Cochrane Database Syst Rev* 3.

Birks JS, Harvey R (2007). Donepezil for dementia due to Alzheimer's disease. Cochrane Dementia and Cognitive Improvement Group. *Cochrane Database Syst Rev* 3.

Black S, Roman GC, Geldmacher DS, Set al.; Donepezil 307 Vascular Dementia Study Group (2003). Efficacy and tolerability of donepezil in vascular dementia: positive results of a 24-week, multicenter, international, randomized, placebo-controlled clinical trial. *Stroke*. 34, 2323–30.

Bodick NC, Offen WW, Levey AI, et al (1997). Effects of xanomeline, a selective muscarinic receptor agonist, on cognitive function and behavioral symptoms in Alzheimer disease. *Arch Neurol* 54, 465–73.

Bonelli SB, Ransmayr G, Steffelbauer M, Lukas T, Lampl C, Deibl M (2004). L-dopa responsiveness in dementia with Lewy bodies, Parkinson disease with and without dementia. *Neurology* 63, 376–8.

Bullock R, Connolly C (2002). Switching cholinesterase inhibitor therapy in Alzheimer's disease: donepezil to rivastigmine, is it worth it? *Int J Geriatr Psychiatry* 17(3), 288–9.

Couratier P, Lesort M, Sindou P, Esclaire F, Yardin C, Hugon J (1996). Modifications of neuronal phosphorylated tau immunoreactivity induced by NMDA toxicity. *Mol Chem Neuropathol* 27, 259–73.

Courtney C, Farrell D, Gray R, et al (2004). Long-term donepezil treatment in 565 patients with Alzheimer's disease (AD2000): randomised double-blind trial. *Lancet* 363, 2105–15.

Cowburn RF, Hardy JA, Roberts PJ (1990). Glutamatergic neurotransmission in Alzheimer's disease. *Biochem Soc Trans* 18, 390–2.

Darreh-Shori T, Almkvist O, Guan ZZ, et al (2002). Sustained cholinesterase inhibition in AD patients receiving rivastigmine for 12 months. *Neurology* 59(4), 563–72.

Degerman Gunnarsson M, Kilander L, Basun H, Lannfelt L (2007). Reduction of phosphorylated tau during memantine treatment of Alzheimer's disease. *Dement Geriatr Cogn Disord* 24(4), 247–52.

Dichgans M, Markus HS, Salloway S, et al (2008). Donepezil in patients with subcortical vascular cognitive impairment: a randomised double-blind trial in CADASIL. *Lancet Neurol* 7(4), 310–8.

Doody R, Wirth Y, Schmitt F, Mobius HJ (2004). Specific functional effects of memantine treatment in patients with moderate to severe Alzheimer's disease. *Dement Geriatr Cogn Disord* 18(2), 227–32.

Emre M, Aarsland D, Albanese A, et al (2004). Rivastigmine for dementia associated with Parkinson's disease. *NEJM* 351, 2509–18.

Erkinjuntti T, Kurz A, Gauthier S, Bullock R, Lilienfeld S, Damaraju CV (2002). Efficacy of galantamine in probable vascular dementia and Alzheimer's disease combined with cerebrovascular disease: a randomized trial. *Lancet* 359, 1283–90.

Esclaire F, Lesort M, Blanchard C, Hugon J. (1997). Glutamate toxicity enhances tau gene expression in neuronal cultures. *J Neurosci Res* 49, 309–18.

Feldman H, Gauthier S, Hecker J, Vellas B, Subbiah P, Whalen E (2001). Donepezil MSAD Study Investigators Group. A 24-week, randomized, double-blind study of donepezil in moderate to severe Alzheimer's disease. *Neurology* 57, 613–20.

Feldman HH, Ferris S, Winblad B, et al (2007). Effect of rivastigmine on delay to diagnosis of Alzheimer's disease from mild cognitive impairment: the InDDEx study Lancet Neurol. *Lancet Neurol* 6(6), 501–12.

Fleischhacker WW, Buchgeher A, Schubert H (1986). Memantine in the treatment of senile dementia of the Alzheimer type. *Prog Neuropsychopharmacol Biol Psychiatry* 10, 87–93.

Förstl H (2000). Clinical issues in current drug therapy for dementia. *Alzheimer Dis Assoc Disord* 14(suppl), S103–8.

Grace J, Daniel S, Stevens T, et al (2001). Long-term use of rivastigmine in patients with dementia with Lewy bodies: an open label trial. *Int Psychogeriatr* 13, 199–205.

Gray CW, Patel AJ (1995). Neurodegeneration mediated by glutamate and β-amyloid peptide: a comparison and possible interaction. *Brain Res* 691, 169–79.

Gu Z, Zhong P, Yan Z (2003). Activation of muscarinic receptors inhibits beta-amyloid peptide-induced signaling in cortical slices. *J Biol Chem* 278, 17546–56.

Hashimoto M, Kazui H, Matsumoto K, et al (2005). Does donepezil treatment slow the progression of hippocampal atrophy in patients with Alzheimer's disease? *Am J Psychiatry* 162, 676–82.

Hock C, Maddalena A, Raschig A, et al (2003). Treatment with the selective muscarinic m1 agonist talsaclidine decreases cerebrospinal fluid levels of A beta 42 in patients with Alzheimer's disease. *Amyloid* 10, 1–6.

Holmes C, Wilkinson D, Dean C, et al (2004). The efficacy of donepezil in the treatment of neuropsychiatric symptoms in Alzheimer disease. *Neurology* 63, 214–9.

Howard RJ, Juszczak E, Ballard CG, et al.; CALM-AD Trial Group (2007). Donepezil for the treatment of agitation in Alzheimer's disease. *N Engl J Med* 357(14), 1382–92.

Kaufer DI, Catt KE, Lopez OL, DeKosky ST (1998). Dementia with Lewy bodies: response of delirium-like features to donepezil. *Neurology* 51, 1512.

Loy C, Schneider L (2007). Galantamine for Alzheimer's disease and mild cognitive impairment. Cochrane Dementia and Cognitive Improvement Group. *Cochrane Database Syst Rev* 3.

Maelicke A (2000). Allosteric modulation of nicotinic receptors as a treatment strategy for Alzheimer's disease. *Dementia* 11(suppl), 11–8.

Mattson MP, Cheng B, Davis D, Bryant K, Lieberburg I, Rydel RE (1992). Beta-amyloid peptides destabilize calcium homeostasis and render human cortical neurons vulnerable to excitotoxicity. *J Neurosci* 12, 376–89.

Mayor S (2005). Regulatory authorities review use of galantamine in mild cognitive impairment. *BMJ* 330(7486), 276.

McKeith I, Del-Ser T, Spano PF, et al (2000). Efficacy of rivastigmine in dementia with Lewy bodies: a randomised, double-blind, placebo controlled international study. *Lancet* 356, 2031–6.

McKeith I, Fairbairn A, Perry R, Thompson P, Perry E (1992). Neuroleptic sensitivity in patients with senile dementia of Lewy body type. *Br Med J* 305, 673–8.

McShane R, Areosa Sastre A, Minakaran N (2007). Memantine for dementia. Cochrane Dementia and Cognitive Improvement Group. *Cochrane Database Syst Rev* 3.

Minett TSC, Thomas A, Wilkinson LM, et al (2003). What happens when donepezil is suddenly withdrawn? An open label trial in dementia with Lewy bodies and Parkinson's disease with dementia. *Int J Geriatr Psychiatry* 18, 988–93.

Orgogozo JM, Rigaud AS, Stoffler A, Mobius HJ, Forette F. (2002). Efficacy and safety of memantine in patients with mild to moderate vascular dementia: a randomised placebo-controlled trial. *Stroke* 33, 1834–9.

Orrell M, Spector A, Thorgrimsen L, Woods B (2005). A pilot study examining the effectiveness of maintenance Cognitive Stimulation Therapy (MCST) for people with dementia. *Int J Geriatr Psychiatry* 20(5), 446–51.

Petersen RC, Thomas RG, Grundman M, et al (2005). Vitamin E and donepezil for the treatment of mild cognitive impairment. *N Engl J Med* 352(23), 2379–88.

Reading PJ, Luce AK, McKeith IG (2001). Rivastigmine in the treatment of parkinsonian psychosis and cognitive impairment: preliminary findings from an open trial. *Mov Disord* 16, 1171–4.

Rockwood K, Fay S, Song X, MacKnight C, Gorman M (2006). Video-Imaging Synthesis of Treating Alzheimer's Disease (VISTA) Investigators. Attainment of treatment goals by people with Alzheimer's disease receiving galantamine: a randomized controlled trial.[see comment]. [Journal Article. Multicenter Study. Randomized Controlled Trial. Research Support, Non-U. S. Gov't] *CMAJ Can Med Assoc J* 174(8), 1099–105.

Rogers SL, Farlow MR, Doody RS, Mohs R, Friedhoff LT; Donepezil Study Group (1998). A 24-week, double-blind, placebo-controlled trial of donepezil in patients with Alzheimer's disease. *Neurology* 50, 136–45.

Rösler M, Anand R, Cicin-Sain A, et al (1999). Efficacy and safety of rivastigmine in patients with Alzheimer's disease: international randomized controlled trial. *BMJ*. 318, 633–8.

Sabbagh M, Hake A, Ahmed S, Farlow M (2005). The use of memantine in dementia with Lewy bodies. *J Alzheimer Dis* 7(4), 285–9.

Sahakian B, Jones G, Levy R, Gray J, Warburton D (1989). The effects of nicotine on attention, information processing, and short-term memory in patients with dementia of the Alzheimer type. *Br J Psychiatry* 154, 797–800.

Shea C, MacKnight C, Rockwood K (1998). Donepezil for treatment of dementia with Lewy bodies: a case series of nine patients. *Int Psychogeriatr* 10, 229–38.

Spector A, Orrell M, Davies S, Woods B (2008). Reality orientation for dementia. Cochrane Dementia and Cognitive Improvement Group. *Cochrane Database Syst Rev* 1.

Spector A, Thorgrimsen L, Woods B, et al (2003). Efficacy of an evidence-based cognitive stimulation therapy programme for people with dementia: randomised controlled trial. *Br J Psychiatry*. 183, 248–54.

Tariot PN, Farlow M, Grossberg G, Graham SM, McDonald S, Gergel I (2004). Memantine treatment in patients with moderate to severe Alzheimer disease already receiving donepezil: a randomized controlled trial. *JAMA* 291(3), 317–24.

Taylor AM, Hoehns JD, Anderson DM, Tobert DG (2002). Fatal aspiration pneumonia during transition from donepezil to rivastigmine. *Ann Pharmacother* 36(10), 1550–3.

Verhoeff NP (2005). Acetylcholinergic neurotransmission and the beta-amyloid cascade: implications for Alzheimer's disease. *Expert Rev Neurother* 5, 277–84.

Wilcock G, Howe I, Coles H, et al (2003). A long-term comparison of galantamine and donepezil in the treatment of Alzheimer's disease. *Drugs Aging* 20(10), 777–89.

Wilcock G, Mobius HK, Stoeffler A (2002). A double-blind placebocontrolled multi-centre study of memantine in mild to moderate vascular dementia (MMM500). *Int Clin Psychopharmacol* 17, 297–305.

Wilkinson D, Doody R, Helme R, et al. (2003). Donepezil in Vascular Dementia. *Neurology* 61, 479–86.

Wilkinson DG, Howe I (2005). Switiching from donepezil to galantamine: a double-blind study of two wash-out periods. *Int J Geriatr Psychiatry* 20, 489–91.

Winblad B, Engedal K, Soininen H, et al (2001). A 1-year, randomized, placebo-controlled study of donepezil in patients with mild to moderate AD. *Neurology* 57, 489–95.

Winblad B, Cummings J, Andreasen N, et al (2007). A six-month double-blind, randomized, placebo-controlled study of a transdermal patch in Alzheimer's disease–rivastigmine patch versus capsule. *Int J Geriatr Psychiatry* 22(5), 456–67.

Winblad B, Kilander L, Eriksson S, et al.; Severe Alzheimer's Disease Study Group (2006). Donepezil in patients with severe Alzheimer's disease: double-blind, parallel-group, placebo-controlled study. *Lancet* 367(9516), 1057–65.

Woods B, Spector A, Jones C, Orrell M, Davies S (2008). Reminiscence therapy for dementia. Cochrane Dementia and Cognitive Improvement Group. *Cochrane Database Syst Rev* 1.

Disease-modifying treatments

7

'Doctor if I take vitamin E, will I prevent Alzheimer's disease?'

The availability of cholinesterase inhibitors (CHEIs) and of the NMDA receptor antagonist memantine is a breakthrough in the treatment of Alzheimer's disease (AD), but they constitute symptomatic treatments and, ultimately, therapies that will be most useful in AD will be disease modifying. Where will such therapies come from? Serendipity is usually the answer, but rationally designed disease-modification strategies are likely to rise out of two broad scientific approaches to understanding AD – molecular pathogenesis and epidemiology. This chapter will review these two approaches, using an update from the original chapter 8 of the first edition of *Management of Dementia*. These dual approaches were also used in a recently re-edited textbook (Bélanger et al, 2007; Launer, 2007).

Possible disease-modification strategies from molecular pathogenesis

The understanding of the pathology of AD, while not complete, can now be described in some detail. The amyloid cascade hypothesis proposed by Hardy and Higgins (1992) stated that amyloid deposition is at the core of AD pathology and that the other pathophysiological features of AD including the accumulation of highly phosphorylated tau in neurofibrillary tangles in neurons, the loss of neurons and the subsequent atrophy and clinical symptoms, all result as a consequence of amyloid deposition. The amyloid cascade hypothesis has had some modifications – it may be intercellular amyloid that is important and it may be necessary for tau to accumulate in tangles (as opposed to this being an epiphenomenon) – but it has nonetheless been substantiated by almost every single important discovery subsequently: all the mutations in different genes that cause early-onset AD result in altered amyloid precursor protein (APP) metabolism and increased amyloid production; the gene associated with late-onset AD, apolipoprotein E (APOE), also binds to and probably affects amyloid; animals harbouring APP mutations, and even more so those with both APP and presenilin-1 mutations, have amyloid deposits and some have cognitive deficits as well. While there are still some unexplained observations, the amyloid cascade hypothesis is the most likely explanation for the pathological events that occur in AD (see Figure 7.1). It is unclear if and how amyloid induces tau phosphorylation; it is possible that tau aggregation could precede phosphorylation

and it is conceivable (and fiercely argued) that amyloid itself may result in cognitive impairment and/or neuronal loss. However, despite these unresolved matters, the scheme shown in Figure 7.1 illustrates most of the disease-modification strategies that have arisen out of the molecular biology of AD.

Altering amyloid

APP is cleaved by at least three secretase activities. Sequential cleavage by β-secretase followed by γ-secretase generates the amyloid moiety, whereas cleavage by α-secretase cuts APP within the amyloid sequence. Each of these enzymes then becomes a target for disease-modifying therapy. Inhibition of β-secretase or γ-secretase would be protective, as would enhancement of the activity of α-secretase. A huge international effort generated a fierce race to discover β-secretase, which was finally revealed in October 1999 and re-named beta-site APP-cleaving enzyme or BACE (Vassar et al, 1999). Inhibitors of this enzyme have been found and examined for therapeutic benefits. γ-Secretase is a more difficult target since it modifies Notch activity, which is involved in haematopoiesis. Inhibition of γ-secretase may well have unwanted and dangerous effects. Nonetheless, inhibitors of γ-secretase are being sought and tested for disease

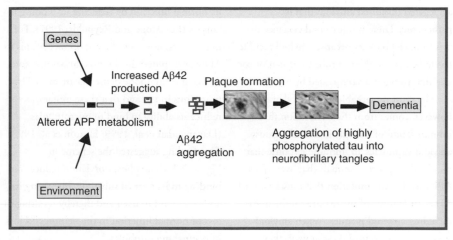

Figure 7.1
The amyloid cascade hypothesis of Alzheimer's disease pathogenesis – each of the steps illustrated is a target for disease modification.

modification. A γ-secretase modulator named tarenflurbil has had encouraging results in phase II (Wilcock et al, 2008) but was non-effective in phase III clinical trials.

Inhibition of an action of an enzyme is generally easier than enhancement of it. However, it is possible that enhancement of the action of α-secretase could be achieved. This enzyme is one of a class that is stimulated by the second messenger, protein kinase C (PKC). Stimulating PKC in cells and animals has been shown to stimulate α-secretase cleavage of APP and in some cases to reduce amyloid production (Racchi et al, 1999). PKC is itself stimulated by a variety of neurotransmitters including certain (m1/m3)

muscarinic receptors. This would suggest that M1 agonists would reduce amyloid and/or increase non-amyloidogenic processing of APP, and indeed in model systems this is exactly what has been found (DeLapp et al, 1998; Nitsch et al, 1996). This exciting finding suggests that any strategy that increases m1 receptor activity, including both m1 agonists and Cholineesterase inhibitors, could have disease-modifying effects.

Finally, it is still not known what is pathogenic about amyloid or, more accurately, in what form is amyloid pathogenic? Is it soluble amyloid peptide, soluble amyloid oligomers or aggregated and fibrillised amyloid? One hypothesis is that it is the aggregated fibrillised amyloid that is pathogenic. There is quite good evidence for this from cell biology because amyloid peptide has to be aged in the test tube to be neurotoxic and this ageing is accompanied by fibrillation.

The most remarkable potential therapy, however, comes from the observation that immunization of transgenic animals against amyloid stimulates an immune response that may be therapeutic. Animals that overexpress APP carrying the mutation that causes familial AD acquire some of the features of the disease including amyloid plaques. When amyloid itself was injected into these animals they developed an immune response and the numbers of plaques dramatically reduced (Schenk et al, 1999). Further work (Bard et al, 2000) shows that passive immunization with antibody has the same effect and that cognitive deficits are reduced. Human clinical trials are under way in AD to establish the safety and efficacy of immunotherapy against amyloid (Wilkinson, 2006).

Targeting tau

The importance of tau to the pathology of dementia came with genetic discoveries (as it so often does). Highly phosphorylated tau, a microtubule-associated protein, essential for normal neuronal functioning, aggregates in neurofibrillary tangles in AD and in other dementias. The phosphorylation of tau reduces its normal function by reducing its binding to tangles (Lovestone and Reynolds, 1997). For many years, however, the importance of this to AD was disputed until it was shown that some forms of frontal-lobe dementia are caused by mutations in tau and that these mutations also reduce its ability to bind to microtubules (Dayanandan et al, 1999; Hutton et al, 1998). This finding suggested the scheme in Figure 7.2 where phosphorylation reduces tau binding to its normal substrate, increasing its ability to bind to itself and thereby resulting in loss of normal function in the neuron and loss of normal microtubules.

Two sites of intervention are suggested by this scheme – prevention of aggregation and prevention of phosphorylation. Tau aggregation inhibitors have not yet been identified but some of the factors that enhance tau aggregation have been demonstrated and such compounds are certainly feasible (Hasegawa et al, 1997). Phosphorylation of tau may be a better or at least more immediate target. Tau is phosphorylated by several enzymes, but we have shown in cells that only one of these is of any good at phosphorylating tau in the same way as in AD brain – an enzyme called GSK-3 (Lovestone et al, 1994). Inhibition of GSK-3 in neurons reduces tau phosphorylation (Hong et al, 1997), suggesting that this may be a feasible strategy. One very strong inhibitor of GSK-3 is known, i.e. lithium. At therapeutic concentrations,

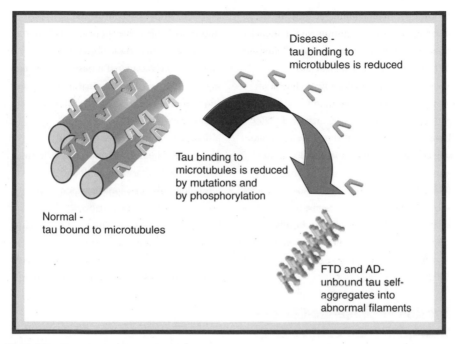

Disease -
tau binding to
microtubules is reduced

Tau binding to
microtubules is reduced
by mutations and
by phosphorylation

Normal -
tau bound to microtubules

FTD and AD-
unbound tau self-
aggregates into
abnormal filaments

Figure 7.2
The formation of paired helical filaments from the microtubule-associated protein tau.

lithium inhibits GSK-3 in neurons, reduces tau phosphorylation and restores the normal function of tau (Hong et al, 1997; Leroy et al, 2000; Lovestone et al, 1999). Two interesting and tantalising consequences arise – could lithium be protective against AD and could this be the action of lithium in bipolar disorder? These are testable suggestions, often asked by patients and relatives.

GSK-3 is also inhibited by PKC and this suggests that activation of PKC would be protective and would reduce tau phosphorylation. We have discussed this above in relation to APP – muscarinic agonists increase PKC activity and increase non-amyloidogenic metabolism. Would the same compounds do the same for tau? Indeed, this appears to be the case and muscarinic agonists reduce tau phosphorylation, do so in non-neuronal cells, neuroblastoma cells and in neurons, and improves the function of tau as they do so (Forlenza et al, 2000; Sadot et al,

1996). Increase in cholinergic function therefore improves cognition, and in model systems, at least, increases non-amyloidogenic APP metabolism and reduces tau phosphorylation. Such a remarkable set of properties suggests a common pathophysiological link (Francis et al, 1999; Lovestone, 1997). Unfortunately, autonomic side effects have limited our ability to use muscarinic agonists as a class of drug (Gauthier, 2001). Clinicopathological studies also indicate that statins may be associated with a reduced burden of neurofibrilliary tangles (Li et al, 2007), but initial clinical trials have been disappointing (e.g. Collins et al, 2002).

Possible disease-modification strategies from epidemiology

Limiting inflammation

It is a curious observation that at the same time that molecular biologists were demonstrating that the immune response generated by amyloid injection may be therapeutic (Schenk et al, 1999), epidemiologists were showing that anti-inflammatory drugs were protective (Andersen et al, 1995; Breitner et al, 1995; Delanty and Vaughan, 1998). These observations were first made in case-control studies that showed that those receiving non-steroidal anti-inflammatory drugs (NSAIDs) for other indications, including leprosy and arthritis, had less AD than

expected. Both case-control and prospective studies with Alzheimer populations have tended to confirm these observations. However, the vaccinated mouse story strongly suggests that not all inflammation is harmful and there may be selective effects, both temporally (i.e., early reduction in inflammation may prevent amyloid generation, late inflammation may help to remove amyloid once formed) and physiologically (i.e., some components of inflammation may be beneficial, others harmful). This may explain in part the failure of all anti-inflammatory clinical trials so far, using selective COX-2 inhibitors as well as traditional NSAIDS (Salloway et al, 2007).

Reducing oxidation

There is a lot of evidence for oxidative stress in AD (Markesbery, 1999; Markesbery and Carney, 1999). Despite the molecular biology and epidemiology advances, age remains the most obvious and important risk factor for AD and oxidative damage is an inevitable consequence of age. Free radicals are generated in most metabolic processes and damage due to free radicals, including lipid peridoxation, increases with age (Butterfield et al, 1999). Amyloid itself may generate free radicals and there is convincing evidence that the toxicity of amyloid, at least in model systems, is reduced by antioxidants (Aksenov et al, 1998). All these data suggest that antioxidants may have disease-modifying effects. Potential antioxidants include vitamin E and vitamin C, idebenone and perhaps MAO-B inhibitors such as selegiline (because MAO-B increases in the free-radical generating astrocytes). Vitamin E has been subjected to clinical trial and shows some beneficial effects in increasing time to nursing home care (Sano et al, 1997). However, the negative results in the study comparing donepezil to tocopherol and placebo in mild cognitive impairment (MCI; Petersen et al, 2005) and a meta-analysis suggesting increased mortality associated with high doses of vitamin E (Miller et al, 2005) has dampened the enthusiasm for this therapeutic approach.

Gingko biloba should be mentioned in this section as it has antioxidant effects. A 42-month placebo-controlled study in cognitively intact subjects did not show a protective effect on progression to Clinical Dementia Rating of 0.5 and memory decline (Dodge et al, 2008), and a large study in the United States over seven years found Gingko Biloba not to be effective in reducing the incidence of dementia (DeKosky et al, 2008).

A final word about the possibility that diet supplementation with fish, fruits and omega-3 rich oils may decrease the risk of AD (Barberger-Gateau et al, 2007), possibly though antioxidant action. Much work remains to be done to determine if lifestyle changes and eating habits need to be altered in individual interested in prevention.

Replacing hormones

Epidemiology studies such as Paganini-Hill and Henderson, 1994, suggested that women receiving hormone replacement therapy were at reduced risk of AD. The biological basis behind such an observation is not known but a variety of plausible suggestions have been made (Birge, 1997). However, it should be noted that not all the epidemiology points in the same direction (Brenner et al, 1994). Despite this, a series of trials have attempted to replace oestrogen as a disease-modifying strategy. The published work was reviewed by Haskell et al (1997) who identified 19 studies including ten randomised trials of replacement therapy. Of these randomised trials, eight claimed therapeutic benefits in memory or attention but did not control for factors such as depression. The study that has had the most negative impact for this therapy was the Women's Health Initiative Memory Study that showed higher risk of MCI and dementia on conjugated equine oestrogens supplementation compared to placebo (Shumaker et al, 2004), negative results confirmed by the COGENT study (Maki et al, 2007).

Reducing vascular disease and diabetes

The distinction between vascular dementia and AD is one of the defining features of the clinical process, but has been challenged by evidence that the distinction between the two conditions may not be as great as once supposed. In fact, mixed dementia may be the most common dementia and is certainly more common than vascular dementia alone (Kalaria & Skoog, 2002; Schneider et al, 2007). Moreover, there is some evidence that vascular risk factors may be independent risk factors for AD (Breteler et al, 1998; Skoog et al, 1999). It follows that prevention of vascular risk factors, such as reducing blood pressure and reducing atherosclereosis, may be of some use in prevention of dementia. Whether the same measures, or others such as aspirin, could have a role in disease modification remains to be seen.

As plasma total homocysteine is a risk factor for vascular disease, it could also be a risk factor for AD or other dementias. Homocysteine levels can be decreased by folate supplementation. A population study suggested a lower risk of AD associated with higher folate intake (Luchsinger et al, 2007) and a placebo-controlled clinical trial with 800 μg daily oral folic acid improved domains of cognitive function (Durga et al, 2007).

Diabetes (Akomolafe et al, 2006) and the metabolic syndrome (Razay et al, 2007) has also been associated with AD. The mechanism whereby diabetes could increase risk is unclear, particularly since insulin resistance is also associated with risk (Kuusisto et al, 1997), suggesting that it is not via the proxy of vascular complications of diabetes (Lovestone, 1999). Because insulin reduces tau phosphorylation (Hong and Lee, 1997) and also increases non-amyloidogenic metabolism of APP (Solano et al, 2000), this suggests that a signalling defect may underlie the association. Effective treatment of diabetes may be disease modifying but only if the signalling cascade is intact. In prospective study showing that diabetes was associated with AD, those patients on insulin actually had higher risk (Ott et al, 1999). This suggests that the association with diabetes shown by epidemiology may be of more use to the molecular biologists looking for new treatments, rather than the public-health clinicians aiming to reduce risk factors. In any case, clinical trials are underway with the anti-diabetic drug rosiglitazone with encouraging results from phase II studies (Watson et al, 2005).

Other treatment strategies

An enormous array of other treatment strategies have been advocated and are been investigated, including trophic factors delivered as small molecules (Longo et al, 2007) or using gene therapy (Tuszynski 2007) and regenerative approaches. Stem cell therapies have perhaps attracted the greatest interest, with recent reports suggesting that implantation of neural stem cells may improve cognition in transgenic mice (Marutle et al, 2007), although this is far more challenging in AD than in Parkinson's disease, and there are considerable practical and scientific barriers to overcome before this becomes a feasible treatment strategy for people with AD. As an alternative, increasing evidence highlights the potential utility of promoting endogenous neurogenesis as a potential treatment strategy (Minger et al, 2007, Greenberg and Jin, 2006), especially as many widely used drugs such as SSRIs enhance stem cell activity (Marcussen et al, 2008).

Disease-modification trial designs

Molecular biology and epidemiology are generating targets for disease modification. But how are attempts to hit these targets be assessed? For a disease in which the person deteriorates relentlessly to distinguish between symptomatic treatment and disease modification is not simple. The first steps in attempts at modification of AD progression, and the scientific measurement of such modification, have been to understand its natural history, and then to develop outcomes appropriate to the stage of disease that is targeted for therapy. Outcomes for early-stage disease are different from those for late-onset disease. Outcomes used have included cognition, function and time to disease stage. Brain imaging has now been added as a valuable surrogate outcome.

The study of the natural history of AD has been facilitated by clinical research criteria

Panel 7.1
Study designs for disease modification

- *parallel groups over 1 year or longer*
- *survival to reach the next milestone(s)*
- *staggered start and withdrawal*
- *single-blind or double-blind active drug withdrawal*
- *open-label extended follow-up*

such as the DSM-IV and the NINCDS-ADRDA criteria (McKhann et al, 1984), which are now being updated to account for the pre-dementia stage of AD (Dubois et al, 2007).

Different clinical trial designs have been proposed to establish disease-modification (Panel 7.1), but it is likely that proof of a true disease-modifying action will require (1) pre-clinical evidence of disease modification, (2) supportive clinical trial observations and (3) supportive biomarker data (Cummings, 2006).

Other points of view about proving disease-modification have been written using consensus among clinicians in Canada (Feldman et al, 2006) and clinicians as well as regulators in Europe (Vellas et al, 2007). The truth is that at this date (Fall, 2008) there has been no successful demonstration of a disease-modifying effect with any compound. Possibly we have selected the wrong stage of AD (when dementia is already clinically apparent).

Summary

- Epidemiology and molecular biology have suggested many targets for therapy. Strategies currently under consideration include decreasing amyloidogenic metabolism or increasing non-amyloidogenic metabolism, reducing amyloid aggregation or reducing tau phosphorylation or aggregation.
- Epidemiology also has suggested targets including anti-inflammatory, hormone replacement, antioxidant and anti-vascular risk strategies.
- Randomised clinical trials of at least 1-year duration are required to test these treatment hypotheses, and will need to be supplemented by strong pre-clinical evidence as well as biological markers.

References

Akomolafe A, Beiser A, Meigs JB, et al (2007). Diabetes mellitus and risk of developing Alzheimer's disease. Results from the Framingham Study. *Arch Neurol* 63, 1551–5.

Aksenov MY, Aksenova MV, Markesbery WR, Butterfield DA (1998). Amyloid β-peptide(1–40)-mediated oxidative stress in cultured hippocampal neurons – protein carbonyl formation, CK BB expression, and the level of Cu, Zn, and Mn SOD mRNA. *J Mol Neurosci* 10, 181–92.

Andersen K, Launer LJ, Ott A, Hoes AW, Breteler MMB, Hofman A (1995). Do nonsteroidal anti-inflammatory drugs decrease the risk for Alzheimer's disease? The Rotterdam Study. *Neurology* 45, 1441–5.

Barberger-Gateau P, Raffaitin C, Letenneur L, et al (2007). Dietary patterns and risk of dementia. The Three-City cohort study. *Neurology* 69, 1921–30.

Bard F, Cannon C, Barbour R, et al (2000). Peripherally administered antibodies against amyloid beta-peptide enter the central nervous system and reduce pathology in a mouse model of Alzheimer disease. *Nat Med* 6, 916–9.

Bélanger S, Pearson V, Poirier J (2007). Pathophysiology: a neurochemical perspective. In: Gauthier S, ed. *Clinical Diagnosis and Management of Alzheimer's Disease*, 3rd edn. London, UK: Informa Healthcare; 15–26.

Birge SJ (1997). The role of estrogen in the treatment of Alzheimer's disease. *Neurology* 48(suppl), S36–41.

Breitner JC, Welsh KA, Helms MJ, et al (1995). Delayed onset of Alzheimer's disease with nonsteroidal anti-inflammatory and histamine H2 blocking drugs. *Neurobiol Aging* 16, 523–30.

Brenner DE, Kukull WA, Stergachis A, et al (1994). Postmenopausal estrogen replacement therapy and the risk of Alzheimer's disease: a population-based case-control study. *Am J Epidemiol* 140, 262–7.

Breteler MMB, Bots ML, Ott A, Hofman A (1998). Risk factors for vascular disease and dementia. *Haemostasis* 28, 167–73.

Butterfield DA, Howard B, Yatin S, et al (1999). Elevated oxidative stress in models of normal brain aging and Alzheimer's disease. *Life Sci* 65, 1883–92.

Collins R, Armitage J, Parish S, Sleight P, Peto R (2002), Heart Protection Study Collaborative Group. MRC/BHF Heart Protection Study of cholesterol lowering with simvastatin in 20536 high-risk individuals: a randomised placebo-controlled trial. *Lancet* 360, 7–22.

Cummings JL (2006). Challenges to demonstrating disease-modifying effects in Alzheimer's disease clinical trials. *Alzheimers Dement* 2, 263–71.

Dayanandan R, Van Slegtenhorst M, Mack TG, et al (1999). Mutations in tau reduce its microtubule binding properties in intact cells and affect its phosphorylation. *FEBS Lett* 446, 228–32.

DeKosky ST, Williamson JD, Fitzpatrick AL, et al (2008). Ginkgo biloba for prevention of dementia: a rondomized controlled trial. *JAMA* 300, 2253–2262.

Delanty N, Vaughan C (1998). Risk of Alzheimer's disease and duration of NSAID use. *Neurology* 51, 652.

DeLapp N, Wu S, Belagaje R, et al (1998). Effects of the M1 agonist xanomeline on processing of human β-amyloid precursor protein (FAD, Swedish mutant) transfected into Chinese hamster ovary m1 cells. *Biochem Biophys Res Commun* 244, 156–60.

Dodge HH, Zitzilberger T, Oken BS, Howieson D, Kaye J (2008). A randomized placebo-controlled trial of Ginkgo Biloba for the prevention of cognitive decline. *Neurology* 70, DOI 10.1212/01.wnl.0000303814.13509.db.

Dubois B, Feldman HH, Jacova C, et al (2007). Research criteria for the diagnosis of Alzheimer's disease: revising the NINCDS-ADRDA criteria. *Lancet Neurol* 6, 734–46.

Durga J, van Boxtel PJ, Schouten EG, et al (2007). Effect of 3-year folic acid supplementation on cognitrive function in older adults in the FACIT trial: a randomized, double blind, controlled trial. *Lancet* 369, 208–16.

Feldman HH, Gauthier S, Chertkow H, Conn DK, Freedman M, MacKnight C; for the 2nd Canadian Conference on Antidementia Guidelines (2006). Canadian guidelines for the development of antidementia therapies: a conceptual summary. *Can J Neurol Sci* 33, 6–26.

Forlenza O, Spink J, Anderton BH, Olesen OF, Lovestone S (2000). Muscarinic agonists reduce tau phosphorylation via GSK-3 inhibition. *J Neural Transm* 107, 1201–12.

Francis PT, Palmer AM, Snape M, Wilcock GK (1999). The cholinergic hypothesis of Alzheimer's disease: a review of progress. *J Neurol Neurosurg Psychiatry* 66, 137–47.

Gauthier S (2001). Muscarinic agonists in Alzheimer's disease. In: Gauthier S, Cummings JL, eds. *Alzheimer's Disease and Related Disorders Annual 2001*. London, UK: Martin Dunitz; 85–96.

Greenberg DA, Jin K (2006) Neurodegeneration and neurogenesis: focus on Alzheimer's disease, current Alzheimer research. 3, 25–8.

Hardy JA, Higgins GA (1992). Alzheimer's disease: the amyloid cascade hypothesis. *Science* 256, 184–5.

Hasegawa M, Crowther RA, Jakes B, Goedert M (1997). Alzheimer-like changes in microtubule-associated protein tau induced by sulfated glycosaminoglycans – inhibition of microtubule binding, stimulation of phosphorylation, and filament assembly depend on the degree of sulfation. *J Biol Chem* 272, 33118–24.

Haskell SG, Richardson ED, Horwitz RI (1997). The effect of estrogen replacement therapy on cognitive function in women: a critical review of the literature. *J Clin Epidemiol* 50, 1249–64.

Hong M, Chen DC, Klein PS, Lee VM (1997). Lithium reduces tau phosphorylation by inhibition of glycogen synthase kinase-3. *J Biol Chem* 272, 25326–32.

Hong M, Lee VMY (1997). Insulin and insulin-like growth factor-1 regulate tau phosphorylation in cultured human neurons. *J Biol Chem* 272, 19547–53.

Hutton M, Lendon CL, Rizzu P, et al (1998). Association of missense and 5'-splice-site mutations in tau with the inherited dementia FTDP-17. *Nature* 393, 702–5.

Kalaria RN, Skoog I (2002). Overlap with Alzheimer's disease. In: Erkinjunti T, Gauthier S, eds. *Vascular Cognitive Impairment*. London, UK: Martin Dunitz; 145–66.

Kuusisto J, Koivisto K, Mykkanen L, et al (1997). Association between features of the insulin resistance syndrome and Alzheimer's disease independently of apolipoprotein E4 phenotype:

cross sectional population based study. *BMJ* 315, 1045–9.

Launer LJ (2007). Pathophysiology: an epidemiological perspective. In: Gauthier S, ed. *Clinical Diagnosis and Management of Alzheimer's Disease*, 3rd edn. London, UK: Informa Healthcare; 27–36.

Leroy K, Menu R, Conreur JL, et al (2000). The function of the microtubule-associated protein tau is variably modulated by graded changes in glycogen synthase kinase-3b activity. *FEBS Lett* 465, 34–38.

Li G, Larson EB, Sonnen JA, et al (2007). Statin therapy is associated with reduced neuropathologic changes of Alzheimer disease. *Neurology* 69, 878–85.

Longo FM, Yang T, Knowles JK, Xie Y, Moore LA, Massa SM (2007). Small molecule neurotrophin receptor ligands: novel strategies for targeting Alzheimer's disease mechanisms. *Curr Alzheimer Res* 4, 503–6.

Lovestone S (1997). Muscarinic therapies in Alzheimer's disease: from palliative therapies to disease modification. *Int J Psychiatr Clin Pract* 1, 15–20.

Lovestone S (1999). Diabetes and dementia: is the brain another site of end-organ damage? *Neurology* 53, 1907–9.

Lovestone S, Davis DR, Webster MT, et al (1999). Lithium reduces tau phosphorylation – effects in living cells and in neurons at therapeutic concentrations. *Biol Psychiatry* 45, 995–1003.

Lovestone S, Reynolds CH (1997). The phosphorylation of tau: a critical stage in neurodevelopmental and neurodegenerative processes. *Neuroscience* 78, 309–24.

Lovestone S, Reynolds CH, Latimer D, et al (1994). Alzheimer's disease-like phosphorylation of the microtubule-associated protein tau by glycogen synthase kinase-3 in transfected mammalian cells. *Curr Biol* 4, 1077–86.

Luchsinger JA, Tang MX, Miller J, Green R, Mayeux R (2007). Relation of higher folate intake to lower risk of Alzheimer disease in the elderly. *Arch Neurol* 64, 86–92.

Maki PM, Gast MJ, Vieweg AJ, Burriss SW, Yaffe K (2007). Hormone therapy in menopausal women with cognitive complaints. *Neurology* 69, 1322–30.

Marcussen AB, Flagstad P, Kristjansen PE, Johansen FF, Englund U (2008). Increase in neurogenesis and behavioural benefit after chronic fluoxetine treatment in Wistar rats. *Acta Neurol Scand* 117, 94–100.

Markesbery WR (1999). The role of oxidative stress in Alzheimer disease. *Arch Neurol* 56, 1449–52.

Markesbery WR, Carney JM (1999). Oxidative alterations in Alzheimer's disease. *Brain Pathology* 9, 133–46.

Marutle A, Ohmitsu M, Nilbratt M, Greig NH, Nordberg A, Sugaya K (2007). Modulation of human neural stem cell differentiation in Alzheimer (APP23) transgenic mice by phenserine. *Proc Natl Acad Sci USA* 104, 12506–11.

McKhann G, Drachman D, Folstein M, Katzman R, Price D, Stadlan EM (1984). Clinical diagnosis of Alzheimer's disease: report of the NINCDS-ADRDA work group under the auspices of Department of Health and Human Services Task Force on Alzheimer's Disease. *Neurology* 34, 939–44.

Miller ER, Pastor-Barriuso R, Dulal D, et al (2005). Meta-analysis: high dosage vitamin E supplementation may increase all-cause mortality. *Ann Intern Med* 142, 37–46.

Minger SL, Ekonomou A, Carta EM, et al (2007). Endogenous neurogenesis in the human brain following cerebral infarction. *Regen Med* 2, 69–74.

Nitsch RM, Wurtman RJ, Growdon JH (1996). Regulation of APP processing – potential for the therapeutical reduction of brain amyloid burden. *Ann N Y Acad Sci* 777, 175–82.

Ott A, Stolk RP, van Harskamp F, Pols HA, Hofman A, Breteler MM (1999). Diabetes mellitus and the risk of dementia: the Rotterdam Study. *Neurology* 53, 1937–42.

Paganini-Hill A, Henderson VW (1994). Estrogen deficiency and risk of Alzheimer's disease in women. *Am J Epidemiol* 140, 256–61.

Petersen RC, Thomas RG, Grundman M, et al (2005). Vitamin E and donepezil for the treatment of mild cognitive impairment. *N Engl J Med* 352(23), 2379–88.

Racchi M, Solano DC, Sironi M, Govoni S (1999). Activity of α-secretase as the common final effector of protein kinase C-dependent and -independent modulation of amyloid precursor protein metabolism. *J Neurochem* 72, 2464–70.

Razay G, Vreugdenhil A, Wilcock G (2007). The metabolic syndrome and Alzheimer disease. *Arch Neurol* 64, 93–6.

Sadot E, Gurwitz D, Barg J, Behar L, Ginzburg I, Fisher A (1996). Activation of m1 muscarinic acetylcholine receptor regulates tau phosphorylation in transfected PC12 cells. *J Neurochem* 66, 877–80.

Salloway S, Mintzer J, Weiner MF, Cummings JL (2007). Disease-modifying therapies in Alzheimer's disease. *Alzheimers Dement* 4, 65–79.

Sano M, Ernesto C, Thomas RG, et al (1997). A controlled trial of selegiline, alpha-tocopherol, or both as treatment for Alzheimer's disease. the Alzheimer's Disease Cooperative Study. *N Engl J Med* 336, 1216–22.

Schenk D, Barbour R, Dunn W, et al (1999). Immunization with amyloid-beta attenuates Alzheimer-disease-like pathology in the PDAPP mouse. *Nature* 400, 173–7.

Schneider JA, Arvanitakis Z, Bang W, Bennett DA (2007). Mixed brain pathologies account for most dementia cases in community-dwelling older persons. *Neurology* 24, 2197–204.

Shumaker SA, Legault C, Kuller L, et al (2004). Conjugated equine oestrogens and incidence of probable dementia and mild cognitive impairment in postmenopausal women: Women's Health Initiative Memory Study. *JAMA* 29, 2947–58.

Skoog I, Kalaria RN, Breteler MMB (1999) Vascular factors and Alzheimer disease. *Alzheimer Dis Assoc Disord* 13(suppl), S106–14.

Solano DC, Sironi M, Bonfini C, Solerte SB, Govoni S, Racchi M (2000). Insulin regulates soluble amyloid precursor protein release via phosphatidyl inositol 3 kinase-dependent pathway. *FASEB J* 14, 1015–22.

Tuszynski MH (2007). Nerve growth factor gene therapy in Alzheimer disease. *Alzheimer Dis Assoc Disord* 21, 179–89.

Vassar R, Bennett BD, Babu-Khan S, et al (1999). Beta-secretase cleavage of Alzheimer's amyloid precursor protein by the transmembrane aspartic protease BACE. *Science* 286, 735–41.

Vellas B, Andrieu S, Sampaio C, Wilcock G; for the European Task Force group (2007). Disease-modifying trials in Alzheimer's disease: a European task force consensus. *Lancet Neurol* 6, 56–62.

Watson GS, Cholerton BA, Reger MA, et al (2005). Preserved cognition in patients with early Alzheimer disease and amnestic mild cognitive impairment during treatment with rosiglitazone: a preliminary study. *Am J Geriatr Psychiatry* 13, 950–8.

Wilcock GK, Black SE, Hendrix SB, Zavitz KH, Swabb EA, Laughlin MA; on behalf of the Tarenflubil Phase II Study investigators (2008). Efficacy and safety of taranflurbil I mild to moderate Alzheimer's disease: a randomized phase II trial. *Lancet Neurol* doi:10.1016/S1474–4422(08)70090–5.

Wilkinson D (2006). Immunotherapy for Alzheimer's disease. In: Gauthier S, Scheltens P, Cummings JL, eds. *Alzheimer's Disease and Related Disorders Annual*, Vol 5. London, UK: Taylor & Francis; 73–88.

Long-term care

'Doctor, does my mother have to go to a nursing home?'

Services for most people with dementia begin and, for many, end in the community. Institutional care is an important part of the overall dementia care and some forms of institutional care prolong the period of time people with dementia can continue to live at home. By supporting carers and providing temporary respite and high quality care, day hospitals and day centres can not only improve the quality of lives of patients and their families but also prolong the period spent in the community. Hospitals themselves can provide respite care periods, which allow the carer some time off whilst also being a period for concentrated attention to the patient's physical health and management of behavioural disturbances can be assessed. The provision of institutional care on a short-term basis to support community care is good practice in that it almost certainly improves quality of life and it is possible that the costs associated with provision of institutional care in the community might reduce the overall costs by limiting the time spent in long-term institutional care, although evidence to support or refute this is hard to find. However, despite the value of community care and short-term institutional care, the provision of long-term institutional care is in many ways the most important element of a service for persons with dementia. Financially, it is the most important element as the largest portion of direct costs for dementia is incurred by services for long-term care. In organisational terms it is the most important factor because long-term care replaces informal care with professional care. But most significantly, entry into long-term care means that families and carers have to come to terms with the last stages of a terminal condition and this point in the process heralds a period of grief and mourning for many relatives. For the patients themselves long-term care usually, although not always, means a loss of autonomy and, all too often, a loss of individuality. Good quality long-term care means many different things from good quality design through to good quality medical care. However, the best quality long-term care should also be attuned to the preservation of dignity and, as far as possible, autonomy of the demented person, and should also preserve the role of the family or principle carer.

Patterns of long-term care

The provision of, and reimbursement for, long-term care differs across countries. In the United Kingdom, older people with mental health problems were, until relatively recently, cared for in large psychiatric hospitals. These institutions were often loathed by the local community and were themselves more often than not housed in the very same buildings as the Victorian Poor Law Workhouses. These institutions were the stuff of Dickens rather than modern dementia service provision and the wards were often of Nightingale design with a central nursing station and beds arrayed down either side of a long high room with windows providing light but no view as they were above the sight line of a seated person. Despite the best efforts of generations of staff, the provision of floral curtains and replacement of beds with easy chairs did little to render these appalling wards suitable for long-term care provision. Over recent years in the United Kingdom, these institutions have all but disappeared and have been replaced by nursing homes, mostly run by for-profit companies or individuals, sometimes not-for-profit organisations and occasionally by the state through social services or health service budgets. A fierce debate has accompanied these changes, often focusing on costs and the sources of income available to fund placement. In the United Kingdom, an attempt has been made to designate long-term care facilities as either providing skilled nursing and medical care or providing partially skilled or non-nursing care. It is immediately obvious that such a division is inherently unstable and to a certain extent arbitrary. It is, however, of real importance as the skilled nursing home care provision is funded by the

National Health Service and therefore free at the point of use and not means-tested, whereas the residential care-only units are funded through social service budgets and means-tested. Given that the value of owner-occupied housing is incorporated into the means testing process (for those without spouses), large numbers of individuals have their estate consumed by long-term care.

In Canada, a similar effect has arisen through a different process as demand for publicly funded institutions outstrips supply and is supplemented by private sector provision. In the United States, the process reaches its natural conclusion as all long-term care is in the private sector. In Scandinavian countries and the Netherlands, by contrast, nursing homes in the community are a well-established component of health care and the process of transfer from hospital to nursing home care has not occurred. As a consequence, small, well-supported, publicly funded nursing homes are a more common feature in these countries (Kane and Kane, 1976).

In addition to the nursing home, many elderly people, some with dementia, live in supported housing – an intermediate form of care which is a compromise between support at home and full institutional care. In the United Kingdom, these most often consist of purpose-built units of 20 to 100 fully independent units with some communal areas. The unit is supported by wardens who may be resident and are most often available 24 hours

a day. In some units, additional care is provided including group activities and meals. Such intermediate care facilities may be able to accommodate those with early dementia and some units have graded levels of accommodation which comprise supported housing, extra-care units and full nursing home provision, thus allowing a person with dementia to move through the system within a single building as the condition deteriorates. Accommodation in supported housing units such as these is often in high demand as the autonomy and privacy of the resident is preserved. For this reason, relatives and other carers are often keen to secure such a placement for their relative with dementia, although the units are most suitable for elderly frail people who are otherwise physically and mentally well. The advice that sheltered accommodation may not be suitable for those with dementia – even in the very early stages – can be a source of conflict. Nonetheless, demand for such placements continues to rise. In the United Kingdom, between 1950 and 1970, the age-specific rate of residency in long-term nursing care facilities rose from 30 to 75 per 1000 (Evans, 1977). Approximately 5% of those older than 65 years live in sheltered accommodation.

In the United States, an intermediate stage between home care support and nursing home care is provided by 'assisted living' units, the fastest-growing sector of long-term care provision (Kopetz et al, 2000). Residents in these units, like those in UK 'extra-care' sheltered accommodation units, are younger, less impaired and suffer less behavioural disturbance than those in nursing home facilities. A similar situation exists in Sweden where 'Group Living' units are increasing in number and provide a level of care intermediate between that of community support and full nursing home care suitable for people with moderate dementia (Annerstedt, 1997).

Predicting entry into long-term care

The decision to place a relative in a long-stay facility is a difficult one and brings with it feelings of guilt and grief as well as more positive aspects such as relief from sleeplessness and respite from behavioural disturbance. The decision of when and whether to enter a nursing home can be a planned decision made by the relative in conjunction with the multidisciplinary team or can occur as the result of a crisis or escalating problems at home. In a small study, Armstrong noted that a number of patients were placed in long-stay care around Christmas time (Armstrong, 2000) and certainly we have noted that for a variety of reasons holiday periods can be particularly stressful. The change in environment, visits from more distant relatives and the general stress and anxiety of such periods can put an extra strain on the carer

and patient and result in a crisis admission. Further evidence that the placement process does not always follow the same set of criteria comes from a study of levels of dependency in a large set of nursing homes where recently placed, low-dependency residents were more likely to be self-funded (as opposed to state funded) than the high-dependency residents, thus indicating that costs and resources also play a role in the decision as to when to enter long-term care (Challis et al, 2000).

Overall characteristics associated with long-term care entry include factors pertaining both to the patient and to the carer. Male carers work differently to female carers and are more likely to access the full range of services on offer in contrast to female carers who tend to be more self- and family reliant. Thus, having a wife may delay entry to a nursing home, while having a husband does so less (Heyman et al, 1997; Tomiak et al, 2000). Spouses make more committed carers than other relatives, the presence of whom increases likelihood of entry to a nursing home (Scott et al, 1997). Hope et al note that factors which predict institutionalisation in the medium term are not the same as factors that precipitate entry to long-term care (Hope et al, 1998), the latter being active behavioural disturbances, in particular aggression. Nonetheless, patients most likely to require long-term care are those with behavioural disturbance, particularly sleeplessness and physical problems including immobility and incontinence (Armstrong, 2000; Hope et al, 1998). A series of systematic and longitudinal studies has found, not surprisingly, that more severely affected patients were admitted to nursing homes but in all cases it appears that it is function and not cognition that best predicts entry (Heyman et al, 1997; Juva et al, 1997; Scott et al, 1997; Severson et al, 1994). In addition to carer factors and patient factors, the availability of other resources delays entry to long-term care (Bianchetti et al, 1995), although in some studies increased provision of services in turn increased the risk of admission to a nursing home probably because service provision reflects both availability and need (Nygaard and Albrektsen, 1992).

Case studies

While the data from surveys such as these is consistent – that more severe, more functionally impaired, older and more physically incapacitated patients are those most likely to be admitted to long-stay care, it can be difficult in practice to predict which individuals (from both the carer and patient perspective) will require nursing home placement. Two examples spring to mind:

Mrs A was referred to specialist services having recently transferred from another family doctor practice. She had not been seen by a doctor for many years. A remarkable story unfurled of a woman who had been living alone and slowly deteriorating first in memory and then in function for more than five years. Her family was very much aware of her plight and arranged a rota so that one of them was with her much of the time and at a very minimum she had two visits a day. All her shopping, cooking and washing needs were provided by her family. She became increasingly disturbed at night and when neighbours complained, members of the family took turns to sleep at her home. This became increasingly difficult for them – they all had families of their own – and the decision was made that Mrs A would go to live with one of her sons. Predictably, she became more confused when she was moved and became sporadically incontinent. The response of her son was to keep her with him at all times. By the time the family sought help, she was accompanying him to work, spending much of the day in the car and was moderately to severely demented with behavioural disturbance (wandering, sleeplessness and occasional vocalisations) as well as being incontinent. The provision of home care supports alleviated the situation somewhat but an extremely difficult situation for the family continued. They continued to refuse long-term care placement.

Ms B on the other hand had mild dementia with no behavioural disturbance and only mild functional impairment. She lived with her friend of many decades who was functionally and cognitively intact. Both women had no family and were independent financially and after much thought requested nursing home placement. Their reasoning was that they could see that they would, over the forthcoming years, become more dependent on the outside world rather than themselves. Although having only mild pathology between them, their lives were already restricted by having to give up driving (for failing eyesight and general nervousness of driving). They felt they would prefer to become accustomed to group living in a caring environment whilst Ms B was able to understand and participate in the decision making.

Both Mrs A and Ms B provided exceptions to the rules predicting entry into nursing home. In fact, such exceptions in our experience are not so uncommon and prove the delights of working with this group of patients and families. Clinicians and services caring for the elderly must be prepared to negotiate with each family as an individual case – for many, entry into long-term care is a devastating and grief-ridden event requiring sensitive support, while for others it can be a rational and life-enhancing process.

Design and long-term care

Any design of a long-term care facility is inevitably a compromise. On the one hand are the requirements of the patient – for the facility to be as like the normal home environment as possible, and on the other hand are the requirements that the facility be manageable – that residents can be seen and be safe. There is the compromise between normal living arrangements (with family, spouse or alone) and the arrangements necessary to provide care (in groups). There is the compromise, as always, between the desirable and the affordable. In the United Kingdom and most developed countries, long-term care facilities are provided both in purpose-built units and in adapted buildings. The latter often have the advantage of being most like the normal housing to which the residents are accustomed. London, for example, is peppered with nursing homes indistinguishable, apart from the sign outside, from the surrounding housing. These facilities, sometimes constructed from internal connections of adjacent housing, are instantly familiar to new residents. The room dimensions and decor are often identical to their own housing, recently vacated. However, these units are often barely suitable for the provision of long-term care to demented patients. The room layout can promote isolation as individual residents spend much time in their own rooms with little scope to move around. Stairs can be narrow and steep and family houses rarely have rooms large enough to accommodate residents in a communal activity with comfort. Purpose-built units on the other hand can offer large and varied communal rooms, easy access and safe environments. On the other hand, they are all too often sterile, institutional and far removed from any environment that the residents have previously lived in.

There are, however, good examples of purpose-built units and designed conversions of existing units that meet the compromise between utility and homeliness. It is this latter characteristic that is so important and the key to homeliness is empathy with the patient. In fact, such empathy is not at all difficult to achieve. As Michael Manser, an architect with a particular interest in design for the infirm, notes, 'What the elderly and disabled probably wanted was what I wanted, but with more comfort, convenience and security ... a location where life can be seen; an opportunity to see and mix with other age groups; a private place to live with your own possessions; and the choice to come and go. A place to live in, not one to wait in and die' (Manser, 1997, p. 411). One of us has a 90-year-old relative in sheltered accommodation. Given a choice between a room overlooking a beautiful and well cared for garden and one on a busy and noisy road next to a shopping centre, she had no hesitation in choosing the latter. As Manser notes, 'Although traditionally the idyllic image for the elderly and demented has been a sylvan scene, they are better stimulated by seeing a busy street scene – the busier the better.'

Manser emphasises the need for long-stay care environments to resemble homes as much as possible despite the presence of protective surfaces, handrails and easy-access doors. This idea has been called the 'homely' concept and is a good guiding principle for long-term care facility design. Alongside the 'homely' concept, long-stay facilities should 'make sense' – for example, corridors that have no purpose other than to be walked down, which people with dementia will do; circular designs will encourage demented people to walk around, surely something unlikely to improve orientation or well-being (Marshall, 1997). As Marshall notes, a corridor retains orientation only to the fire exit. Orientation can be aided by good design; constructive use of textures to differentiate a throughway from a bedroom (vinyl vs. carpet for example) and different color schemes for bathrooms, living rooms and bedrooms are both techniques used to good effect in some homes. Bedrooms need to have enough space to accommodate personal effects and residents should be encouraged to bring in their own furniture, mirrors and pictures even if this compromises the overall design of the building.

This personalisation of space should continue through to the staff. All too often the people in a home become the residents. Not the same thing at all. Staff need to be helped and encouraged to find the person behind the resident, to learn something of their personal history, likes and dislikes and their family. All too often this is not the case and it can be difficult to identify a locus of responsibility for ensuring that staff not only care for but actually recognise the people in the home. As Cooper notes, 'Old people admitted to long-term care in the homes are in a real sense displaced persons . . . biographical data that might be used to take advantage of former skills and interests are usually missing or fragmentary; the residents have lost their shadows.' (Cooper, 1997). Good design as well as good staff morale and training could help preserve this individuality.

Dementia management in long-term care

A well-functioning long-stay facility will undertake regular medical and psychiatric review of residents. Health care issues in congregate dwellings include attention to group health (e.g. provision of influenza immunisation) as well as individual health. Much physical disability goes unrecognised in long-term care; large rates of undiagnosed hypotension were found in one study, for example (Butler et al, 1999) a problem that can increase morbidity and indeed mortality through falls. The abilities of individual residents should be known by the staff in order that maximisation of their cognitive and functional status can be achieved. Given that those in long-term care tend to be more impaired and more behaviourally disturbed, there is considerable need for good management of behavioural disturbance, mindful of the fact that these are the individuals most vulnerable to side effects and the more serious adverse consequences of

psychotropic drug, especially antipsychotics (discussed in chapter 2).

Importantly, traditional approaches to care have often ignored the social world of the person with dementia, their own experiences of the process which they were going through, their previous skills and coping strategies. In the early 1990s, psychosocial theories and treatments began to emerge, which have been collectively termed 'the new culture of care'. The term 'person-centered care' is used to define the work involving the carer–client relationship, in which the carer sees the person first and the diagnosis of dementia as secondary. The focus of being person-centred is defined by Kitwood (1997) as ' . . . a standing or status that is bestowed upon one human being, by others, in the context of relationship and social being. It implies recognition, respect and trust'. Kitwood translated the philosophy into a more practical focus on 'positive person work', in which he identified the particular skills a practitioner needed to promote and achieve person-centred practice: recognition, negotiation, collaboration, fun, celebration, relaxation, validation and holding and facilitation. Building on the principles of person-centred care, it is clear that much more individualised approach is needed to meet people's needs appropriately. This includes more flexible and individually tailored provision of activities tailored to the preferences and abilities of the individual and a more flexible approach to the

24-hour needs of people with dementia (Train et al 2005). This type of approach is geared towards maximising the quality of life for a particular individual and will probably also play an important role in preventing the emergence of psychiatric and behavioural symptoms.

Much behavioural disturbance in homes is, in fact, a direct consequence of some form of care activity, particularly aspects of personal such as washing and dressing (Keatinge et al, 2000). Often thoughtful care planning and good interpersonal skills will reduce fear, misunderstanding and the consequent behavioural manifestations. Controlled trials in this area have highlighted that a structured assessment of unmet needs can be extremely helpful in better meeting needs and improving care plans (Orrell et al, 2007). Specific therapeutic approaches that have been shown to be effective are individualised music therapy sessions, which reduce agitation (Gerdner, 2000); physical activity and exercise, which improves health, reduces deterioration in mobility and function and improves mood (Lazowski et al, 1999; Teri et al, 2003). Other activities such as reminiscence therapy (Livingston et al, 2005) and positive individualised activities also have a significant beneficial impact upon mood (Teri et al, 1997). The use of biographical information and carer discussions can play a key role in generating a programme in developing an individualised and effective care plan. Even

with the best care, a substantial proportion of residents will display such disturbance regardless of stimulation. Active management of behavioural disturbance is therefore a priority in care homes and the principles outlined in chapter 2 are as applicable in a nursing home as at home. In the United States and elsewhere, some nursing homes have specialised in providing dementia care, known in the United States as special care units (SCUs). Alongside this development was the directive in the United States (Omnibus Reconciliation Act of 1987 [OBRA-87]) that encouraged reduced use of physical restraints and antipsychotic medication. Many assumed that if SCUs do indeed provide better care, then this would be manifested in lower use of psychotropic medications and physical restraints. However, this does not appear to be the case as shown in a survey of such homes in four states. Physical restraint was similar in SCUs but the use of antipsychotic medication was both common and actually higher in SCUs (52% of patients compared to 34–38% in the other units [Phillips et al, 2000). It is difficult to know whether the higher use of psychotropic medication in SCUs reflects more efficacious treatment of BPSD, higher rates of behavioural and psychological symptoms of dementia (BPSD) or whether staff in SCUs have lower thresholds for using psychotropic medication. Good management of BPSD should not avoid the use of psychotropic medication – it is an effective and evidence-based treatment of a distressing set of symptoms – but there is no excuse for continued treatment beyond the necessary. Good practice within long-term care facilities would ensure regular review of all medication and audit of use over time in order to identify trends. In one such audit, we found increased use of psychotropic medication correlated with decreased numbers of staff on duty at night for example (unpublished observation). Specific non-pharmacological and pharmacological interventions for the management of BPSD are reviewed in detail in chapter 2.

The key issue in providing high quality person-centred care and the effective non-pharmacological management of BPSD is the training received by the nursing and care staff within care and nursing home settings. There are only minimal training requirements, not usually including mandatory training in dementia care in most countries. This often means that care staff are undertaking a very difficult job without the necessary training and support to undertake the task effectively. Controlled trials indicate that training can significantly improve care (Burgio et al, 2002) and reduce antipsychotic use without any deterioration of behaviour (Fossey et al, 2006). This type of comprehensive evidence-based approach is, however, rarely implemented in usual clinical or care practice (Alzheimer's Society, 2007), and it is important for specialist services to contribute to overall training and support in care homes and nursing homes as well as providing a consultancy service for individual patients.

Particularly, as dementia becomes more severe, meeting the physical health needs of individuals becomes even more difficult. This is not only important with respect to the health of individuals but also to their well-being, and physical illness is a common trigger for behavioural symptoms. One specific issue is pain, which is difficult to assess in people with more severe dementia. Generally, pain is under-treated, and recent excellent work from the Cohen-Mansfield group reports methods for assessing pain and demonstrates the benefits of more proactive analgesia (Cohen-Mansfield and Lipson 2008). In end-stage dementia swallowing, skin and joint care, fluid and nutrition intake, tackling end-of-life issues and proving appropriate support for families, requires a range of skills and multi-disciplinary team working. New nursing strategies are being developed to improve quality of care in the severe stage of AD (Sandman et al, 2007).

Summary

- Many but not all people with dementia spend some time in a long-term care facility.
- Patient features that predict entry to long-term care include severity of functional impairment and behavioural disturbance as well as incontinence and physical immobility.

- Carer characteristics increasing likelihood of admission to a nursing home include being male.
- No two carer and patient dyads are alike, however, and some patients require early admission whilst others strenuously defer admission.
- The time of admission to a long-term care facility is difficult for the carer, the wider family and the patients themselves. This stage requires sensitive handling and support.
- Good homes incorporate good design. Good design is homely. The requirements of patients with dementia are not so dissimilar from yours.
- Individualised and person-centred care, provided by well-trained and well-supported staff are the key elements of high-quality, long-term care provision.
- The needs of residents include regular medical review, individually tailored activities and appropriate management of behavioural disturbance.

References

Alzheimer's Society (UK) (2007). Dementia Care in Care Homes.

Annerstedt L (1997). Group-living care: an alternative for the demented elderly. *Dement Geriatr Cogn Disord* 8, 136–42.

Armstrong M (2000). Factors affecting the decision to place a relative with dementia into residential care. *Nurs Stand* 14, 33–7.

Bianchetti A, Scuratti A, Zanetti O, et al (1995). Predictors of mortality and institutionalization in Alzheimer disease patients 1 year after discharge from an Alzheimer dementia unit. *Dementia* 6, 108–12.

Burgio LD, Stevens A, Burgio KL, Roth DL, Paul P, Gerstle J (2002). Teaching and maintaining behavior management skills in the nursing home. *Gerontologist* 42, 487–96.

Butler R, Fonseka S, Barclay L, et al (1999). The health of elderly residents in long term care institutions in New Zealand. *N Z Med J* 112, 427–9.

Challis D, Mozley CG, Sutcliffe C, et al (2000). Dependency in older people recently admitted to care homes. *Age Ageing* 29, 255–60.

Cohen-Mansfield J, Lipson S (2008). The utility of pain assessment for analgesic use in persons with dementia. *Pain* 134, 16–23.

Cooper B (1997). Principles of service provision in old age psychiatry. In: Jacoby R, Oppenheimer C, eds. *Psychiatry in the elderly*, 1 edn. Oxford: Oxford University Press; 357–75.

Evans JG (1977). Current issues in the United Kingdom. In: Exton-Smith AN, Evans JG, ed. *Care of the Elderly: Meeting the challenge of dependency*. New York: Grune and Stratton; 128–46.

Fossey J, Ballard C, Juszczak E, et al (2006). Effect of enhanced psychosocial care on antipsychotic use in nursing home residents with severe dementia: cluster randomised trial. *BMJ* 332, 756–61.

Gerdner LA (2000). Effects of individualized versus classical 'relaxation' music on the frequency of agitation in elderly persons with Alzheimer's disease and related disorders. *Int Psychogeriatr* 12, 49–65.

Heyman A, Peterson B, Fillenbaum G, et al (1997). Predictors of time to institutionalization of patients with Alzheimer's disease: The CERAD experience 17. *Neurology* 48, 1304–9.

Hope T, Keene J, Gedling K, et al (1998). Predictors of institutionalization for people with dementia living at home with a carer. *Int J Geriatr Psychiatry* 13, 682–90.

Juva K, Makela M, Sulkava R, et al (1997). One-year risk of institutionalization in demented outpatients with caretaking relatives. *Int Psychogeriatr* 9, 175–82.

Kane RL, Kane RA (1976). *Long-term care in six countries.* Washington, DC: Department of Health, Education and Welfare.

Keatinge D, Scarfe C, Bellchambers H, et al (2000). The manifestation and nursing management of agitation in institutionalised residents with dementia. *Int J Nurs Pract* 6, 16–25.

Kitwood T (1997). *Dementia reconsidered.* Buckingham: Open University Press.

Kopetz S, Steele CD, Brandt J, et al (2000). Characteristics and outcomes of dementia residents in an assisted living facility. *Int J Geriatr Psychiatry* 15, 586–93.

Lazowski DA, Ecclestone NA, Myers AM, et al (1999). A randomized outcome evaluation of group exercise programs in long-term care institutions. *J Gerontol A Biol Sci Med Sci* 54, M621–8.

Livingston G, Johnston K, Katona C, Paton J, Lyketsos CG (2005). Old Age Task Force of the World Federation of Biological Psychiatry. Systematic review of psychological approaches to the management of neuropsychiatric symptoms of dementia. *Am J Psychiatry* 162, 1996–2021.

Manser M (1997). Better quality environments for people with dementia – design of environments. In: Jacoby R, Oppenheimer C, eds. *Psychiatry in the elderly,* 2nd edn. Oxford: Oxford Unversity Press; 410–20.

Marshall M (1997). Better quality environments for people with dementia – design and technology for people with dementia. In: Jacoby R, Oppenheimer C, eds. *Psychiatry in the elderly,* 2nd edn. Oxford: Oxford Unversity Press; 421–35.

Nygaard HA, Albrektsen G (1992). Risk factors for admission to a nursing home. A study of elderly people receiving home nursing. *Scand J Prim Health Care* 10, 128–33.

Orrell M, Hancock G, Hoe J, Woods B, Livingston G, Challis D (2007). A cluster randomised controlled trial to reduce the unmet needs of people with dementia living in residential care. *Int J Geriatr Psychiatry* 22, 1127–34.

Phillips CD, Spry KM, Sloane PD, et al (2000). Use of physical restraints and psychotropic medications in Alzheimer special care units in nursing homes. *Am J Public Health* 90, 92–6.

Sandman PO, Edvardson D, Winblad B (2007). Care of patients in the severe stage of dementia. In: Gauthier S, ed. *Clinical diagnosis and management of Alzheimer's disease.* London: Informa Healthcare; 233–46.

Scott WK, Edwards KB, Davis DR, et al (1997). Risk of institutionalization among community long-term care clients with dementia. *Gerontologist* 37, 46–51.

Severson MA, Smith GE, Tangalos EG, et al (1994). Patterns and predictors of institutionalization in community- based dementia patients. *J Am Geriatr Soc* 42, 181–5.

Teri L, Gibbons LE, McCurry SM, et al (2003). Exercise plus behavioral management in patients with Alzheimer disease: a randomized controlled trial. *JAMA* 290, 2015–22.

Teri L, Logsdon RG, Uomoto J, McCurry SM (1997). Behavioral treatment of depression in dementia patients: a controlled clinical trial. *J Gerontol B Psychol Sci Soc Sci* P159–66.

Tomiak M, Berthelot JM, Guimond E, et al (2000). Factors associated with nursing-home entry for elders in Manitoba, Canada. *J Gerontol A Biol Sci Med Sci* 55, M279–87.

Train G, Nurock S, Kitchen G, Manela M, Livingston G (2005). A qualitative study of the views of residents with dementia, their relatives and staff about work practice in long-term care settings. *Int Psychogeriatr* 17, 237–51.

Assessment scales in the management of Alzheimer's disease

The core of all assessment in dementia care is careful enquiry and attentive listening, and there is no substitute for a clinical interview by a trained doctor, nurse, psychologist, occupational therapist or social worker. However, having acknowledged this, there is a special and important role for the use of formal scales in dementia assessment. The reason for this is not entirely clear – assessment scales are used in all medical conditions in research but only rarely elsewhere in ordinary clinical practice. Probably the reasons are multiple: partly because the patients themselves are less able to describe the symptoms, partly because the symptoms are context sensitive (better functional ability in own home than in somewhere less familiar, for example) and partly because the symptoms are, to a certain extent, subjective. Some types of symptoms lend themselves better to formal assessment using scales than others. Cognitive symptoms in particular lend themselves so readily to assessment using scales that for many clinicians it is easy to forget that the widespread use of scales in clinical practice is a relatively recent phenomenon. Assessing other aspects of the life and symptoms of a person with dementia is more challenging.

One advantage of using scales is that of reliability both between assessors and over the course of time. Another is the reductionism itself: although this has to be balanced by a clinical and 'holistic' assessment, the provision of a number allows measurement of change and ready comparison of the patient to others and to population norms. One further, almost hidden, advantage of scales is that they can act as a prompt to full clinical assessment. The incorporation of a set of assessment scales into clinical practice can encourage, for example, full and pro-active assessment of behaviour rather than relying on a reactive assessment following carer complaint.

When planning an assessment using scales, it is important to balance practicality with scientific rigor. Scales formulated for use in research may not always be suitable for use in clinical practice. One example of this that has caused particular problems is that of cognitive tests. Invariably, clinical trials of cholinesterase inhibitors have used the ADAS-cog (Rosen et al, 1984) as a primary outcome measure, in the mild-to-moderate stages of Alzheimer's disease (AD). The scale is comprehensive enough to give an assessment of a wide range of cognitive abilities, is specifically designed for assessment of cognitive function and is highly reliable with excellent validity. However, it takes approximately 45 minutes with a trained rater. Few clinical services have the resources to contemplate such an assessment in routine clinical practice. On the

other hand, the Mini-Mental State Examination (MMSE, Folstein et al, 1975) is a relatively non-comprehensive measure of cognitive function that was designed for screening for cognitive impairment rather than actual assessment, but can be completed in 10 minutes and has well-established thresholds. Moreover, it is almost certainly the most widely used scale measuring any aspect of dementia; it has extensive normative data in the elderly available and must be familiar to almost all of us working in the clinical field of dementia care. Therefore, when choosing a scale to measure cognition in response to drug treatments in clinical practice, the choice is between the excellent scale used as the primary outcome measure in clinical trials that takes longer than the time available for full assessment of the patient, and a less than perfect scale that is easily performed. The choice is obvious for most and we imagine few services use the ADAS-cog.

In this chapter we have included a selection of scales that we hope might be useful in clinical practice. Most scales, including these, were derived with research in mind and all have received at least some form of validity and reliability testing. Most but not all of these scales are useful for research – many are indeed used in clinical studies but the needs of research are such that the choice of a particular scale for a particular project carries quite different considerations to choosing a scale for clinical practice. We increasingly use scales, including some of those below; in our clinical practice and for use in this context the scale should be relatively quick to perform and should require minimal training to conduct it and to interpret the results. The use of self-rating scales by carers complements interviewer assessment. Preferably, the scale will be used with ease by all members of the multi-disciplinary team.

Assessment of cognition

Three levels of assessment can be distinguished with respect to cognition. Comprehensive measures of cognitive ability, assessment or screening in secondary care and screening in primary care. Comprehensive measures of cognitive ability are best performed using scales all the way from the ADAS-cog through a detailed neuropsychometric testing taking many hours. We include the ADAS-cog (Rosen et al, 1984) as it may have some role in memory clinics and other specialized units and has been extremely widely used in clinical trials. For other purposes, the MMSE is most suitable for screening in primary and secondary care, although there are limitations to its use as noted above. These limitations are not always appreciated. For example, the U.K. expert group the National Institute for Clinical Excellence (NICE), a government-established body, approved the use of cholinesterase inhibitors for AD only for those with MMSE scores between 20 and 10. However, clearly it is possible to have dementia, and to be recognized as having dementia, with a score above 20, and clinical trial evidence clearly indicates that these individuals benefit from treatment with a cholinesterase inhibitor. The problem is rigid application and interpretation, and not the scale itself. As with all tests, the MMSE should be used to complement and not to replace clinical assessment. The MMSE is a 30-point scale with 24 being the cut-off for screening for dementia and takes 10 minutes or less to perform with only a minimal amount of training necessary. This is a screening instrument and not a diagnostic test, and the cut-off is variable depending upon a number of factors including education. In addition, the score of the same individual can vary 2 or 3 points over a couple of days (Bowie et al, 1999). Providing the test is interpreted with common sense, and in the context of the overall history and assessment, it is a valuable part of a clinical evaluation. The clock drawing test can also be used as a fairly coarse measure of deterioration, and methods of rating have been developed to provide better standardization (e.g. Brodaty & Moore, 1997). CLOX takes this further in a two-stage clock drawing assessment involving free drawing in the presence of visual distractors on the assessment sheet, followed by clock copying, and has the advantage of a good correlation with both MMSE and executive performance (Royall et al, 1998). The

Montreal Cognitive Assessment (MoCA) is a brief cognitive assessment that is substantially more sensitive for the identification of mild cognitive impairment and mild AD than the MMSE (Nasreddine et al, 2005), and may also be a sensitive method for assessing cognitive impairment in people with Parkinson's disease and stroke. For the assessment of people with severe dementia, the Severe Impairment Battery (SIB, Saxton et al, 1990) is a 100-point assessment, taking approximately 30 minutes to complete. The scale is user-friendly and sensitive to change so that it can be very useful for assessing and measuring treatment response in these individuals. Clearly, short assessment scales cannot replace a detailed neuropsychological evaluation, but standardized assessments of key cognitive domains such as executive function (e.g. EXIT 25; Royall et al, 1992) and memory (e.g., the Word list tasks from the ADAS-cog; Rosen et al, 1984) may be helpful at the bedside or in the clinic.

Assessment of behavioural and psychological symptoms of dementia

Assessment of behaviour has only recently come under the scrutiny of the advocates of scales. While there are many scales that measure different aspects of behaviour, there is one scale in particular that has been used to good effect in both clinical practice and clinical research. The Neuro-psychiatric

Inventory (NPI) is a brief clinician-conducted interview with a carer that takes 10 minutes and rates the extent, severity and frequency of a variety of behaviours. It is an excellent and deservedly popular scale. A specific nursing home version is available, but it is important to ensure that the member of staff knows the resident well and is a reliable informant. Assessing depression in dementia is particularly difficult, and the NPI can usefully be complemented by the Cornell Depression in Dementia Scale (CDDS; Alexopoulos et al, 1988). The Cohen-Mansfield Agitation Inventory (Cohen-Mansfield et al, 1989) is an excellent and more comprehensive assessment specifically for agitation and aggression. Other more specialized scales for individual BPSD symptoms are listed in Panel 9.1.

Assessment of function

We have recommended three scales of assessment of function. This was a somewhat arbitrary and personal choice as there are many scales in this area. The Alzheimer's Disease Cooperative Study-Activities of Daily Living Inventory (ADCS-ADL) scale was systematically refined into a well-validated, 27-item informant scale with good inter-rater and test–re-test reliability, which has been widely used in clinical trials (Galasko et al, 1997). The Bristol Activities of Daily Living scale (B-ADL), which has been used in several longitudinal clinical studies and a few clinical trials, is more detailed and covers a broader range of disability, which may be advantageous in long-term follow-up studies (Bucks et al, 1996). The Disability Assessment in Dementia (DAD; Gelinas et al, 1999) is a 40-question scale designed to be completed by interviewing the carer regarding instrumental and self-care activities performed during the previous two weeks, widely used in ongoing disease-modifying trials in AD.

Global assessment and carer assessment

It was probably the FDA decision to require a global deterioration measure in assessing efficacy of anti-dementia drugs that has resulted in the huge importance attached to this aspect of assessment. We include details of two overlapping assessment measures. The Clinicians' Global Impression of Change and its variants (e.g. Schneider et al, 1997) are used in almost all clinical trials and are essentially a formalisation of the clinicians' assessment of change based upon their assessment of the patient together and in some cases with the carers' assessment. The Functional Assessment Staging (FAST, Reisberg, 1988) assesses the severity of dementia based on a broad range of domains including function and language, and has the advantage of providing good sensitivity even in the more severe stages of dementia. For follow-up of treatment over a year or more, the Clinical Dementia Rating (CDR) scale is widely used and is useful, exploring in a semi-structured way the six complementary domains of cognition and function, the method of summing the boxes developed as part of the CERAD initiative increases the reliability (Fillenbaum et al, 1996). The CDR is less useful than the FAST for people with severe dementia.

Assessment of carer stress is of two broad types – assessment of the carer's mental state using generic stress or depression scales, or assessment of the carer's perceptions of the amount of time spent caring or the burden they are suffering from. We have included one scale we find useful, the Zarit Burden Interview. This is a self-report scale, now available in a shortened form, which is probably more helpful for clinical practice (Bedard et al, 2001).

Quality of life

The ultimate goal of most clinical interventions for people with dementia is to improve quality of life, yet this is rarely measured in clinical trials or clinical practice. Although there are inherent difficulties in evaluating quality of life in people with dementia, simple scales such as the QOL-AD, combining a patient and informant report, are simple to administer and appear to be reliable (Logsdon et al, 2002). The recently developed DEMQOL (Smith et al, 2007) is more detailed, and may have advantages but has yet to be fully validated. Dementia Care Mapping (DCM) is a more labour-intensive method,

Table 9.1
Listing of some additional scales that may be helpful in the assessment of unmet need or specific BPSD symptoms

BPSD Symptom	Scale	Comment
Anxiety	RAID (Shankar et al, 1999)	The only validated scale specifically to measure anxiety in people with dementia
Psychosis	CUSPAD (Devanand et al, 1992)	Useful scale evaluating a range of specific psychotic symptoms
Agitation	CMAI (Cohen-Mansfield et al, 1989)	Useful and comprehensive scale that is sensitive to change and a good method to evaluate treatment response
Aggression	RAGE (Patel & Hope, 1992)	Useful aggression assessment for in-patients or people residing in a care home, designed to be completed by nursing staff
Apathy	Apathy scale (Starkstein et al, 1995)	The NPI provides an evaluation of apathy, but this is a useful scale if a more detailed assessment is needed
Comprehensive overall rating of BPSD	PBE (Hope & Fairburn, 1992)	Lengthy and detailed evaluation taking an hour or more to complete, but provides the most comprehensive overall assessment of BPSD.
Unmet need	CANE (Reynolds et al, 2000)	A validated assessment of unmet needs that is particularly useful in planning care for people in nursing homes.

Readers interested in these and other scales in old-age psychiatry can consult the compendium of scales put together by Burns et al (2004).

allowing up to six people with dementia in care homes, attending daycare settings or admitted to in-patient units to be evaluated simultaneously over a 6-hour period of daytime observation (Kitwood & Bredin, 1997). Wellbeing, social withdrawal and activities are measured, providing useful proxies of quality of life (Fossey et al, 2002), and the scale can also be used to measure the quality of a care environment (Ballard et al, 2001) or as a medium for audit and practice development (Brooker, 2005).

Other scales

A range of other potentially useful scales for specific BPSD symptoms, comprehensive overall evaluation of BPSD and for assessing unmet needs are given in Table 9.1. In addition, a list of recent, highly recommended scales can be found in the following list:

Highly Recommended New Scales

ADCS-ADL: Alzheimer's Disease Cooperative Study-Activities of Daily Living

Galasko D. *Alzheimer Disease & Associated Disorders*, Vol. 11, Suppl 2, (Appendix III), 1997.

CMAI: Cohen-Mansfield Agitation Inventory

Galasko D. *Alzheimer Disease & Associated Disorders*, Vol. 11, Suppl 2, (Appendix III), 1997.
Assessment Scales in Old Age Psychiatry, Second Edition; (Burns A, Lawlor B, Craig S, eds.),
London: Martin Dunitz, 2007, p. 159.

SWE-TOOL

Sandman PO. Care of patients in the severe stage of dementia. In: *Clinical Diagnosis and
Management of Alzheimer's Disease, Third Edition*; (Gauthier S, ed.), London: Informa UK Ltd.,
2006, pp 243–244.

QOL-AD: Quality of Life in Alzheimer's Disease

Logsdon RG. In: *Assessment Scales in Old Age Psychiatry, Second Edition*; (Burns A, Lawlor B,
Craig S, eds.), London: Martin Dunitz, 2007, pp 232–234.

MoCA: Montreal Cognitive Assessment

Nasreddine Z. In: *Clinical Diagnosis and Management of Alzheimer's Disease, Third Edition*,
(Gauthier S, ed.), London: Informa UK Ltd., 2007, p. 207.

CLOX: Clock drawing task

Royall DR, Cordes JA, Polk M. CLOX: an executive clock drawing task. J Neurol Neurosurg Psychiatry,
1998(64):588–594.

Royall DR. Executive control function in mild cognitive impairment and Alzheimer's disease.
In: *Alzheimer's Disease and Related Disorders Annual 5* (Gauthier S, Scheltens P, Cummings
JL, eds.), London: Taylor & Francis, 2005, pp 35–62.

Mini-Mental State Examination (MMSE)

Max   *Score*
score

ORIENTATION
5   ( )   *What is the (year) (season) (date) (month) (day)?*
5   ( )   *Where are we: (state) (county) (town) (hospital) (floor)?*

REGISTRATION
3   ( )   *Name 3 objects: (1 second to say each). Then ask the patient all three after you have said*
              them.
              Give 1 point for each correct answer. Then repeat them until the patient learns all 3. Count
              trials and record.
              Number of Trials _____

ATTENTION AND CALCULATION
5   ( )   *Serial 7's. 1 point for each correct. Stop after 5 answers. If the patient refuses, spell "world"*
              backwards.

RECALL
3   ( )   *Ask for 3 objects repeated above. Give 1 point for each correct.*

LANGUAGE
9   ( )   *Name a pencil; name a watch. (2 points)*
              Repeat the following: "No ifs, ands or buts." (1 point)
              Follow a three stage command: "Take this paper in your right hand, fold it in half, and put
              it on the floor." (3 points)
              Read and obey the following: "Close your eyes." (1 point)

              Write a sentence. (1 point)

              Copy a design. (1 point)

Total Score _____   *Assess level of*   _____
                        consciousness   *Alert   Drowsy   Stupor   Coma*
                        along a continuum

Reprinted from the *Journal of Psychiatric Research*, Vol. 12, Folstein MF, Folstein SE. McHugh PR "Mini-Mental State": a practical method for grading the cognitive state of patients for the clinician. (1975), with permission from Elsevier Science.

Mental Test Score (MTS)/Abbreviated Mental Test Score

ORIGINAL TEST ITEMS	
	Score
Name	*0/1*
Age	*0/1*
Time (to nearest hour)	*0/1*
Time of day	*0/1*
Name and address for five minutes recall; this should be repeated by the patient to ensure it has been heard correctly.	
Mr John Brown	*0/1/2*
42 West Street	*0/1/2*
Gateshead	*0/1*
Day of week	*0/1*
Date (correct day of month)	*0/1*
Month	*0/1*
Year	*0/1*
Place: Type of place (i.e. Hospital)	*0/1*
Name of Hospital	*0/1*
Name of ward	*0/1*
Name of town	*0/1*
Recognition of two persons (doctor, nurse, etc.)	*0/1/2*
Date of birth (day and month sufficient)	*0/1*
Place of birth (town)	*0/1*
School attended	*0/1*
Former occupation	*0/1*
Name of wife, sib or next of kin	*0/1*
Date of First World War (year sufficient)	*0/1*
Date of Second World War (date sufficient)	*0/1*
Name of present Monarch	*0/1*
Name of present Prime Minister	*0/1*
Months of year backwards	*0/1/2*
Count 1–20	*0/1/2*
Count 20–1	*0/1/2*
Total	*(34)*

ABBREVIATED MENTAL TEST SCORE

1. *Age*
2. *Time (to nearest hour)*
3. *Address for recall at end of test – this should be repeated by the patient to ensure it has been heard correctly: 42 West Street*
4. *Year*
5. *Name of hospital*
6. *Recognition of two persons (doctor, nurse, . . .)*
7. *Date of birth*
8. *Year of First World War*
9. *Name of present Monarch*
10. *Count backwards 20–1*

(each question scores one mark)

Source: Hopkinson M (1972) Evaluation of a mental test score for assessment of mental impairment in the elderly. *Age and Ageing* 1: 233–8. By kind permission of Oxford University Press.

Alzheimer's Disease Assessment Scale (ADAS) – Cognitive and Non-Cognitive Sections (ADAS-Cog, ADAS-Non-Cog)

Cognitive Items

1. Spoken language ability _____
2. Comprehension of spoken language _____
3. Recall of test instructions _____
4. Word-finding difficulty _____
5. Following commands _____
6. Naming: objects, fingers _____

High:	1	2	3	4	Fingers: Thumb
Medium:	1	2	3	4	Pinky Index
Low:	1	2	3	4	Middle Ring

7. Constructions: drawing _____

   Figures correct: 1   2   3   4

   Closing in: Yes _____ No _____
8. Ideational praxis _____

   Step correct:

   1   2   3   4   5
9. Orientation _____

   Day ___ Year ___ Person ___ Time of day ___

   Date ___ Month ___ Season ___ Place ___
10. Word recall: mean error score _____
11. Word recognition: mean error score _____

    Cognition total _____

Non-cognitive Items (all rated by examiner)

12. Tearful _____
13. Appears/reports depressed mood _____
14. Concentration, distractibility _____
15. Uncooperative to testing _____
16. Delusions _____
17. Hallucinations _____
18. Pacing _____
19. Increased motor activity _____
20. Tremors _____
21. Increase/decrease appetite _____

    Noncognition total _____

Total Scores

Cognitive behavior _____

Non-cognitive behavior _____

Word recall _____

Word recognition _____

Total _____

Rating: x = not assessed

0 = not present

1 = very mild

2 = mild

3 = moderate

4 = moderately severe

5 = severe

Spoken language – quality of speech not quantity.
Comprehension – do not include responses to commands.
Do not include finger or object naming.

Score 0–5 steps correct

1–4 steps correct

2–3 steps correct

3–2 steps correct

4–1 steps correct

5 – cannot do one step correct

Name fingers of dominant hand and high/medium/low frequency objects.

0 = all correct; one finger incorrect and/or one object incorrect

1 = two–three fingers and/or two objects incorrect

2 = two or more fingers and three–five objects incorrect

3 = three or more fingers and six–seven objects incorrect

4 = three or more fingers and eight–nine objects incorrect

Ability to copy circle, two overlapping rectangles, rhombus and cube.

5 components in sending self a letter

1 = difficulty or failure to perform one component

2 = difficulty and/or failure to perform two components

3 = difficulty and/or failure to perform three components

4 = difficulty and/or failure to perform four components

5 = difficulty and/or failure to perform five components

Date, month, year, day of week, season, time of day, place and person.

Noncognitive behavior is evaluated over preceding week to interview.

American Journal of Psychiatry, Vol. 141, pp. 1356–64, 1984. Copyright 1984, the American Psychiatric Association. Reprinted by permission.

Clock Drawing Test

A priori criteria for evaluating clock drawings
(10 = best and 1 = worst)

10–6. *Drawing of Clock Face with Circle and Numbers is Generally Intact*

10. *Hands are in correct position (i.e. hour hand approaching 3 o'clock)*

9. *Slight errors in placement of the hands*

8. *More noticeable errors in the placement of hour and minute hands*

7. *Placement of hands is significantly off course*

6. *Inappropriate use of clock hands (i.e. use of digital display or circling of numbers despite repeated instructions)*

5–1. *Drawing of Clock Face with Circle and Numbers is Not Intact*

5. *Crowding of numbers at one end of the clock or reversal of numbers. Hands may still be present in some fashion.*

4. *Further distortion of number sequence. Integrity of clock face is now gone (i.e. numbers missing or placed at outside of the boundaries of the clock face).*

3. *Numbers and clock face no longer obviously connected in the drawing. Hands are not present.*

2. *Drawing reveals some evidence of instructions being received but only a vague representation of a clock.*

1. *Either no attempt or an uninterpretable effort is made.*

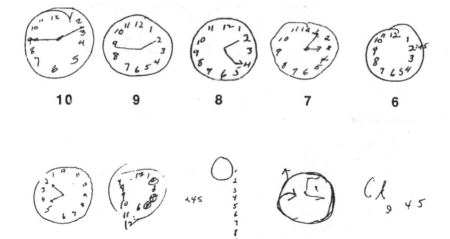

Samples of clock drawings from Alzheimer patients with evaluations of best (10) to worst (1).

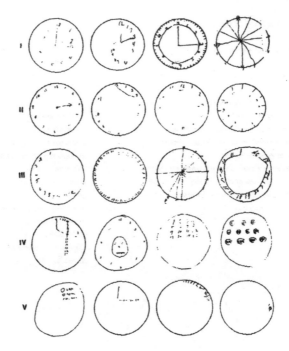

Clinical examples of clock errors

Classification of clock errors

I   *Visuospatial*

(a)   *Mildly impaired spacing of times*

(b)   *Draws times outside circle*

(c)   *Turns page while writing numbers so that some numbers appear upside down*

(d)   *Draws in lines (spokes) to orient spacing*

II   *Errors in denoting the time as 3 o'clock*

(a)   *Omits minute hand*

(b)   *Draws a single line from 12 to 3*

(c)   *Writes the words '3 o'clock'*

(d)   *Writes the number 3 again*

(e)   *Circles or underlines 3*

(f)   *Unable to indicate 3 o'clock*

III   *Visuospatial*

(a)   *Moderately impaired spacing of times (so that 3 o'clock cannot be accurately denoted)*

(b) *Omits numbers*

Preservation

(a) *Repeats the circle*

(b) *Continues on past 12 to 13, 14, 15, etc.*

Right–Left reversal – numbers drawn counterclockwise

Dygraphia – unable to write numbers accurately

IV *Severely disorganized spacing*

(a) *Confuses 'time' – writes in minutes, times of day, months or seasons*

(b) *Draws a picture of human face on the clock*

(c) *Writes the word 'clock'*

V *Unable to make any reasonable attempt at a clock*
  (excludes severe depression or other psychotic state)

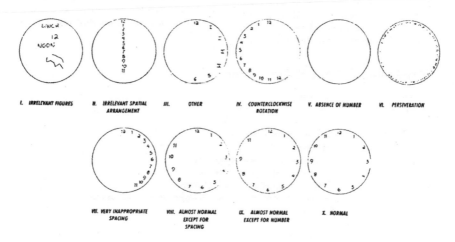

The 10 clock patterns

Sources: Sunderland T, Hill JL, Mellow AM, Lawlor BA, Gundersheimer J, Newhouse PA, Grafman JH (1989) Clock drawing in Alzheimer's disease; and Wolf-Klein GR, Silverstone FA, Levy AP, Brod MS, Breuer J (1989) Screening for Alzheimer's disease by clock drawing, *Journal of American Geriatrics Society.* Vol. 37, no. 8. pp. 725–9 and 730–4, respectively; also Brodaty H, Moore CM (1997) The Clock Drawing Test for dementia of the Alzheimer's type: a comparison of three scoring methods in a memory disorders clinic; and Shulman K, Shedleksky R, Silver I (1986) The challenge of time. Clock drawing and cognitive function in the elderly, *International Journal of Geriatric Psychiatry.* Vol. 12, pp. 619–27 and Vol. 1, pp. 135–40, respectively (Copyright John Wiley & Sons Limited. Reproduced with permission).

Severe Impairment Battery (SIB)

Reference   Saxton J, McGonigle-Gibson K, Swihart A, Miller M, Boller F (1990) Assessment of severely impaired patients: description and validation of a new neuropsychological test battery. *Psychological Assessment* 2: 298–303

Time taken   30–40 minutes (reviewer's estimate)
Rating   by trained interviewer

Main indications
Assessment of cognitive function, particularly in severe dementia.

Commentary
The Severe Impairment Battery (SIB) has the strength of assessing cognitive function in patients with moderate to severe dementia. Items are single words or one-step commands combined with gestures. Nine areas are assessed (see below), and the score is between 0 and 100. It appears to change. Panisset et al (1994)

examined 69 patients with severe dementia using the SIB and found it to be a helpful neuropsychological measure in people with severe dementia.

Additional references
Albert M, Cohen C (1992) The Test for Severe Impairment, an instrument for the assessment of patients with severe cognitive dysfunction. *Journal of American Geriatric Society* 40: 449–53.
Panisset M, Roudier M, Saxon J et al (1994) Severe Impairment Battery: a neuropsychological battery for severely impaired patients. *Archives of Neurology* 51: 41–5.

Severe Impairment Battery Domains

Domain	Questions
Orientation	*Name*
	Place (town)
	Time (month and time of day)
Attention	*Digit span*
	Counting to visual and auditory stimuli
Language	*Auditory and reading comprehension*
	Verbal fluency (food and months of the year)
	Naming from description, pictures of objects, objects, colors and forms
	Repetition
	Reading
	Writing
	Copying of written material
Praxis	*How to use a cup, a spoon*
Visuospatial	*Discrimination of colors and forms*
Construction	*Spontaneous drawing, copying and tracing a figure*
Memory	*Immediate short- and long-term recall for examiner's name, objects, colors, forms and a short sentence*
Orientation to name	*When the patient's name is called from behind*
Social interaction	*Shaking hands, following general direction*

Source: Panisset M, Roudier M, Saxton J et al (1994) Severe Impairment Battery: a neuropsychological battery for severely impaired patients. *Archives of Neurology* 51: 41–5.

BEHAVE-AD

Part 1: Symptomatology
Assessment Interval: Specify: _____ wks.
Total Score: _____

a.   Paranoid and Delusional Ideation

1.   "People are Stealing Things" Delusion

0 = Not present.

1 = Delusion that people are hiding objects.

2 = Delusion that people are coming into the home and hiding objects or stealing objects.

3 = Talking and listening to people coming into the home.

2.   "One's House is Not One's Home" Delusion

0 = Not present.

1 = Conviction that the place in which one is residing is not one's home (e.g. packing to go home; complaints, while at home, of "take me home").

2 = Attempt to leave domiciliary to go home.

3 = Violence in response to attempts to forcibly restrict exit.

3.   "Spouse (or Other Caregiver) is an Imposter" Delusion

0 = Not present.

1 = Conviction that spouse (or other caregiver) is an imposter.

2 = Anger toward spouse (or other caregiver) for being an imposter.

3 = Violence towards spouse (or other caregiver) for being an imposter.

4.   "Delusion of Abandonment" (e.g. to an Institution)

0 = Not present.

1 = Suspicion of caregiver plotting abandonment or institutionalization (e.g. on telephone).

2 = Accusation of a conspiracy to abandon or institutionalize.

3 = Accusation of impending or immediate desertion or institutionalization.

5.   "Delusion of Infidelity"

0 = Not present.

1 = Conviction that spouse and/or children and/or other caregivers are unfaithful.

2 = Anger toward spouse, relative, or other caregiver for infidelity.

3 = Violence toward spouse, relative, or other caregiver for supposed infidelity.

6.   "Suspiciousness/Paranoia" (other than above)

0 = Not present.

1 = Suspicious (e.g. hiding objects that he/she later may be unable to locate).

2 = Paranoid (i.e. fixed conviction with respect to suspicions and/or anger as a result of suspicions).

3 = Violence as a result of suspicions.

Unspecified?

Describe

7.   Delusions (other than above)

0 = Not present.

1 = Delusional.

2 = Verbal or emotional manifestations as a result of delusions.

3 = Physical actions or violence as a result of delusions.

Unspecified?

Describe

b.   Hallucinations

8.   Visual Hallucinations

0 = Not present.

1 = Vague: not clearly defined.

2 = Clearly defined hallucinations of objects or persons (e.g. sees other people at the table).

3 = Verbal or physical actions or emotional responses to the hallucinations.

9.   Auditory Hallucinations

0 = Not present.

1 = Vague: not clearly defined.

2 = Clearly defined hallucinations of words or phrases.

3 = Verbal or physical actions or emotional response to the hallucinations.

10. Olfactory Hallucinations

0 = Not present.

1 = Vague: not clearly defined.

2 = Clearly defined.

3 = Verbal or physical actions or emotional responses to the hallucinations.

11. Haptic Hallucinations

0 = Not present.

1 = Vague: not clearly defined.

2 = Clearly defined.

3 = Verbal or physical actions or emotional responses to the hallucinations.

12. Other Hallucinations

0 = Not present.

1 = Vague: not clearly defined.

2 = Clearly defined.

3 = Verbal or physical actions or emotional responses to the hallucinations.

Unspecified?

Describe

c.   Activity Disturbances

13. Wandering: Away From Home or Caregiver

0 = Not present.

1 = Somewhat, but not sufficient to necessitate restraint.

2 = Sufficient to require restraint.

3 = Verbal or physical actions or emotional responses to attempts to prevent wandering.

14. Purposeless Activity (Cognitive Abulia)

0 = Not present.

1 = Repetitive, purposeless activity (e.g. opening and closing pocketbook, packing and unpacking clothing, repeatedly putting on and removing clothing, opening and closing drawers, insistent repeating of demands or questions).

2 = Pacing or other purposeless activity sufficient to require restraint.

3 = Abrasions or physical harm resulting from purposeless activity.

15. Inappropriate Activity

0 = Not present.

1 = Inappropriate activities (e.g. storing and hiding objects in inappropriate places, such as throwing clothing in wastebasket or putting empty plates in the oven; inappropriate sexual behavior, such as inappropriate exposure).

2 = Present and sufficient to require restraint.

3 = Present, sufficient to require restraint, and accompanied by anger or violence when restraint is used.

d.   Aggressiveness

16. Verbal Outbursts

0 = Not present.

1 = Present (including unaccustomed use of foul or abusive language).

2 = Present and accompanied by anger.

3 = Present, accompanied by anger, and clearly directed at other persons.

17. Physical Threats and/or Violence

0 = Not present.

1 = Threatening behavior.

2 = Physical violence.

3 = Physical violence accompanied by vehemence.

18. Agitation (other than above)

0 = Not present.

1 = Present.

2 = Present with emotional component.

3 = Present with emotional and physical component.

Unspecified?

Describe

e.   Diurnal Rhythm Disturbances

19. Day/Night Disturbance

0 = Not present.

1 = Repetitive wakenings during night.

2 = 50% to 75% of former sleep cycle at night.

3 = Complete disturbance of diurnal rhythm (i.e. less than 50% of former sleep cycle at night).

f. Affective Disturbance

20. Tearfulness

0 = *Not present.*

1 = *Present.*

2 = *Present and accompanied by clear affective component.*

3 = *Present and accompanied by affective and physical component (e.g. "wrings hands" or other gestures).*

21. Depressed Mood: Other

0 = *Not present.*

1 = *Present (e.g. occasional statement "I wish I were dead," without clear affective concomitants).*

2 = *Present with clear concomitants (e.g. thoughts of death).*

3 = *Present with emotional and physical component (e.g. suicide gestures).*

Unspecified?

Describe

g. Anxieties and Phobias

22. Anxiety Regarding Upcoming Events (Godot Syndrome)

0 = *Not present.*

1 = *Present: Repeated queries and/or other activities regarding upcoming appointments and/or events.*

2 = *Present and disturbing to caregivers.*

3 = *Present and intolerable to caregivers.*

23. Other Anxieties

0 = *Not present.*

1 = *Present.*

2 = *Present and disturbing to caregivers.*

3 = *Present and intolerable to caregivers.*

Unspecified?

Describe

24. Fear of Being Left Alone

0 = *Not present.*

1 = *Present: Vocalized fear of being alone.*

2 = *Vocalized and sufficient to require specific action on part of caregiver.*

3 = *Vocalized and sufficient to require patient to be accompanied at all times.*

25. Other Phobias

0 = *Not present.*

1 = *Present.*

2 = *Present and of sufficient magnitude to require specific action on part of caregiver.*

3 = *Present and sufficient to prevent patient activities.*

Unspecified?

Describe

Part 2: Global Rating

With respect to the above symptoms, they are of sufficient magnitude as to be:

0 = *Not at all troubling to the caregiver or dangerous to the patient.*

1 = *Mildly troubling to the caregiver or dangerous to the patient.*

2 = *Moderately troubling to the caregiver or dangerous to the patient.*

3 = *Severely troubling or intolerable to the caregiver or dangerous to the patient.*

Neuropsychiatric Inventory (NPI)

Reference   Cummings JL, Mega M, Gray K, Rosenberg-Thompson S, Carusi DA, Gornbein J (1994)
The Neuropsychiatric Inventory: comprehensive assessment of psychopathology in dementia.
Neurology 44: 2308–14

Time taken   10 minutes
Rating   by clinician in interview with a carer

Main indications
The Neuropsychiatric Inventory (NPI) evaluates a wider range of psychopathology than comparable instruments, and may help distinguish between different causes of dementia; it also records severity and frequency separately.

Commentary
The NPI is a relatively brief interview assessing 10 behavioural disturbances: delusions; hallucinations; dysphoria; anxiety; agitation/aggression; euphoria; disinhibition; irritability/ lability; apathy; and aberrant motor behavior. It uses a screening strategy to cut down the length of time the instrument takes to administer, but it obviously takes longer if replies are positive. It is scored from 1 to 144. Severity and frequency are independently assessed. The authors reported on 40 caregivers, and content and concurrent validity and inter-rater and test/retest reliability were assessed. Some 45 assessments were used for the inter-rater reliability and 20 for

test/retest reliability. Concurrent validity was found to be satisfactory using a panel of appropriated experts; concurrent reliability was determined by comparing the NPI subscale with subscales of the BEHAVE-AD (page 75) and the Hamilton Depression Rating Scale (page 4). Highly significant correlations were found. A high level of internal consistency (0.88) was found using a Cronbach's coefficient. Inter-rater reliability revealed agreement in over 90 ratings, and test/retest reliability (a second interview within 3 weeks) was very highly significant. A training pack and further information is available from the author.

Address for correspondence
JL Cummings
Neurobehavior Unit
Psychiatry Service (116F)
West Los Angeles, VAMC
11301 Wilshire Blvd
Los Angeles
CA 90073
USA

Neuropsychiatric Inventory (NPI)

Description of the NPI

The NPI consists of 12 behavioral areas

Delusions	*Apathy*
Hallucinations	*Disinhibition*
Agitation	*Irritability*
Depression	*Aberrant motor behavior*
Anxiety	*Night-time behaviors*
Euphoria	*Appetite and eating disorders*

Frequency is rated as
1. *Occasionally – less than once per week*
2. *Often – about once per week*
3. *Frequently – several times a week but less than every day*
4. *Very frequently – daily or essentially continuously present*

Severity is rated as
1. *Mild – produce little distress in the patient*
2. *Moderate – more disturbing to the patient but can be redirected by the caregiver*
3. *Severe – very disturbing to the patient and difficult to redirect*

Distress is scored as
0 — no distress
1 — minimal
2 — mild
3 — moderate
4 — moderately severe
5 — very severe or extreme

For each domain there are 4 scores. Frequency, severity, total (frequency × severity) and caregiver distress. The total possible score is 144 (i.e. A maximum of 4 in the frequency rating × 3 in the severity rating × 12 remaining domains). This relates to changes, usually over the 4 weeks prior to completion.

Source: Cummings JL, Mega M, Gray K, Rosenberg-Thompson S, Carusi DA, Gornbein J (1994) The Neuropsychiatric inventory: comprehensive assessment of psychopathology in dementia. *Neurology* 44: 2308–14.

Cornell Scale for Depression in Dementia

A.   *Mood-Related Signs*
1.   *Anxiety*
     anxious expression, ruminations, worrying
2.   *Sadness*
     sad expression, sad voice, tearfulness
3.   *Lack of reactivity to pleasant events*
4.   *Irritability*
     easily annoyed, short tempered

B.   *Behavioral Disturbance*
5.   *Agitation*
     restlessness, handwringing, hairpulling
6.   *Retardation*
     slow movements, slow speech, slow reactions
7.   *Multiple physical complaints*
     (score 0 if GI symptoms only)
8.   *Loss of interest*
     less involved in usual activities (score only if change occurred acutely, i.e. in less than 1 month)

C.   *Physical Signs*
9.   *Appetite loss*
     eating less than usual
10. *Weight loss*
     (score 2 if greater than 5 lb in 1 month)

11. *Lack of energy*
     fatigues easily, unable to sustain activities (score only if change occurred acutely, i.e. in less than 1 month)

D.   *Cyclic Functions*
12. *Diurnal variation of mood*
     symptoms worse in the morning
13. *Difficulty falling asleep*
     later than usual for this individual
14. *Multiple awakenings during sleep*
15. *Early morning awakening*
     earlier than usual for this individual

E.   *Ideational Disturbance*
16. *Suicide*
     feels life is not worth living, has suicidal wishes, or makes suicide attempt
17. *Poor self-esteem*
     self-blame, self-depreciation, feelings of failure
18. *Pessimism*
     anticipation of the worst
19. *Mood-congruent delusions*
     delusions of poverty, illness, or loss

Rating:
a = Unable to evaluate; 0 = Absent; 1 = Mild or intermittent; 2 = Severe
All based on week prior to interview

Reprinted by permission of Elsevier Science, Inc. from Cornell Scale for Depression in Dementia by George S. Alexopoulos, Robert C. Abrams, Robert C. Young, and Charles A. Shamoian, *Biological Psychiatry*, Vol. 23, pp. 271–84. Copyright © 1988 by The Society of Biological Psychiatry.

Interview for Deterioration in Daily Living Activities in Dementia (IDDD)

Reference   Teunisse S, Derix MMA (1991) Measuring functional disability in community dwelling dementia patients: development of a questionnaire. *Tijdschrift voor Gerontologie en Geriatrie* **22**: 53–9

Time taken   15 minutes (reviewer's estimate)
Rating   by interview with main caregiver

Main indications
To assess activities of daily living in dementia.

Commentary
The scale covers 33 activities such as washing, dressing, and eating as well as more complex activities such as shopping, writing and answering the telephone, tasks performed equally by men and women (earlier scales of activities of daily living tended to rely more heavily on female-dominated and less complex tasks). Both the initiative to perform activities and the performance itself were evaluated. There was high internal consistency (alpha = 0.94) and two groups of items were discriminated: those related to self-care activity and those to more complex tasks. Functioning of the patient is examined in a structured verbal interview with the carer. The scoring is rated on a three-point scale: 1 where help is almost never needed or there has been no change, 2 where help is sometimes needed or when help is needed more often than previously, and 3 when help is almost always needed or help is needed much more than previously. The scoring is carried out by referring to behaviour in the last month, comparing it with how it was before the onset of the dementia. After a negative response the questioner is asked to check that the behaviour is unchanged compared with what it was like previously, and after positive response questions are asked: "is the help really necessary?" "what happens if you don't help?" and "do you have to help more often than before?"

The original paper rated functional disability along with cognitive impairment (measured by the CAMCOG), behavioural disturbances [measured by the GIP (page 124)] and carer burden [measured by an instrument related to the Zarit Burden Interview (page 239)]. Inter-relationships were found in 30 mild to moderately impaired patients with dementia. Functional disability was strongly related to cognitive deterioration and behavioural disturbances, and moderately related to burden experienced by carers. Since 1991, the IDDD has been translated into several languages and a paper-and-pencil version has been used in the measurement of treatment effects.

Additional reference
Teunisse S, Derix MMA, van Crevel H (1991) Assessing the severity of dementia: patient and caregiver. *Archives of Neurology* **48**: 274–7.

Address for correspondence
S Teunisse
Psychology Department
William Guild Building
King's College
University of Aberdeen
Aberdeen AB24 2UB
UK

Interview for Deterioration in Daily Living Activities in Dementia (IDDD)

1. *Do you have to tell her that she should wash herself (take the initiative to wash herself; not only washing of hands or face, but also washing of whole body)?* 1 2 3 8 9
2. *Do you have to assist her in washing (finding face cloth, soap; soaping and rinsing of the body)?* 1 2 3 8 9
3. *Do you have to tell her that she should dry herself (take the initiative to dry herself, for example looking or fetching for the towel)?* 1 2 3 8 9
4. *Do you have to assist her in drying (drying individual body-parts)?* 1 2 3 8 9
5. *Do you have to tell her that she should dress herself (take the initiative to dress herself, for example walking to the wardrobe)?* 1 2 3 8 9
6. *Do you have to assist her in dressing herself (putting on individual clothes in right order)?* 1 2 3 8 9
7. *Do you have to assist her in doing up her shoes, using zippers or buttons?* 1 2 3 8 9
8. *Do you have to tell her that she should brush her teeth or comb her hair?* 1 2 3 8 9
9. *Do you have to assist her in brushing her teeth?* 1 2 3 8 9
10. *Do you have to assist her in combing her hair?* 1 2 3 8 9
11. *Do you have to tell her that she should eat (take the initiative to eat; in case eating is elicited by others, it should be asked if she would take the initiative spontaneously)?* 1 2 3 8 9
12. *Do you have to assist her in preparing a slice of bread?* 1 2 3 8 9
13. *Do you have to assist her in carving meat, potatoes?* 1 2 3 8 9
14. *Do you have to assist her in drinking or eating?* 1 2 3 8 9
15. *Do you have to tell her that she should use the lavatory (take the initiative to go to the lavatory when necessary)* 1 2 3 8 9
16. *Do you have to assist her in using the toilet (undressing herself, using toilet, using closet paper)?* 1 2 3 8 9
17. *Do you have to assist her in finding her way in the house (finding different rooms)?* 1 2 3 8 9
18. *Do you have to assist her in finding her way in familiar neighbourhood outside the house?* 1 2 3 8 9
19. *Does she – as often as before – take the initiative shopping (take the initiative to figure out what is needed)?* 1 2 3 8 9
20. *Do you have to assist her in shopping (finding her way in the shops; getting goods in needed quantity)?* 1 2 3 8 9
21. *Do you – or the shop-assistant – have to tell her that she should pay?* 1 2 3 8 9
22. *Do you – or the shop-assistant – have to assist her in paying (knowing how much she should pay and how much should be reimbursed)?* 1 2 3 8 9
23. *Is she – as often as before – interested in newspaper, book or post?* 1 2 3 8 9
24. *Do you have to assist her in reading (understanding written language)?* 1 2 3 8 9
25. *Do you have to assist her in writing a letter or card, or completing a form (writing of more than one sentence)?* 1 2 3 8 9
26. *Does she – as often as before – start a conversation with others?* 1 2 3 8 9
27. *Do you have to assist her in expressing herself verbally?* 1 2 3 8 9

28. *Does she – as often as before – pay attention to conversation by other people?* 1 2 3 8 9
29. *Do you have to assist her in understanding spoken language?* 1 2 3 8 9
30. *Does she – as often as before – take the initiative to use the phone (both answering the phone and calling someone)?* 1 2 3 8 9
31. *Do you have to assist her in using the phone (both answering the phone and calling someone)?* 1 2 3 8 9
32. *Do you have to assist her in finding things in the house?* 1 2 3 8 9
33. *Do you have to tell her to put out gas or coffee machine?* 1 2 3 8 9

Rating:
1 = (nearly) no help needed/no change in help needed
2 = sometimes help needed/help more often needed
3 = (nearly) always help needed/help much more often needed
8 = no evaluation possible
9 = not applicable

Reproduced (with permission from the American Medical Association) from Teunisse S et al. (1991) Assessing the severity of dementia: patient and caregiver. *Archives of Neurology*, **48**: 274–7. Copyright 1991. American Medical Association.

Bristol Activities of Daily Living Scale

Reference Bucks RS, Ashworth DL, Wilcock GK, Siegfried K (1996) Assessment of activities of daily living in dementia: development of the Bristol Activities of Daily Living Scale. *Age and Ageing* 25: 113–20

Time taken 15 minutes (reviewer's estimate)
Rating by carer

Main indications
Assessment of activities of daily living in patients with dementia either in the community or on clinical research trial.

Commentary
The scale was designed specifically for use in patients with dementia, and consists of 20 daily living abilities. Face validity was measured by way of carer agreement that the items were important, construct validity was confirmed by principal components analysis, concurrent validity by assessment with observed performance and good test/rest reliability. Three phases in the design of the

scale were described. Anyone designing a scale should read this to serve as a model of clarity.

Additional reference
Patterson MB, Mack JL, Neundorfer MM et al (1992) Assessment of functional ability in Alzheimer's disease: a review and preliminary report on the Cleveland Scale for Activities of Daily Living. *Alzheimer Disease and Associated Disorders* 6: 145–63.

Address for correspondence
GK Wilcock
Department of Care of the Elderly
Frenchay Hospital
Bristol BS16 1LE
UK

Bristol Activities of Daily Living Scale

1. Food
a. Selects and prepares food as required   [ ]
b. Able to prepare food if ingredients set out   [ ]
c. Can prepare food if prompted step by step   [ ]
d. Unable to prepare food even with prompting and supervision   [ ]
e. Not applicable   [ ]

2. Eating
a. Eats appropriately using correct cutlery   [ ]
b. Eats appropriately if food made manageable and/or uses spoon   [ ]
c. Uses fingers to eat food   [ ]
d. Needs to be fed   [ ]
e. Not applicable   [ ]

3. Drink
a. Selects and prepares drinks as required   [ ]
b. Can prepare drinks if ingredients left available   [ ]
c. Can prepare drinks if prompted step by step   [ ]
d. Unable to make a drink even with prompting and supervision   [ ]
e. Not applicable   [ ]

4. Drinking
a. Drinks appropriately   [ ]
b. Drinks appropriately with aids, beaker/straw etc.   [ ]
c. Does not drink appropriately even with aids but attempts to   [ ]
d. Has to have drinks administered (fed)   [ ]
e. Not applicable   [ ]

5. Dressing
a. Selects appropriate clothing and dresses self   [ ]
b. Puts clothes on in wrong order and/or back to front and/or dirty clothing   [ ]
c. Unable to dress self but moves limbs to assist   [ ]
d. Unable to assist and requires total dressing   [ ]
e. Not applicable   [ ]

6. Hygiene
a. Washes regularly and independently   [ ]
b. Can wash self if given soap, flannel, towel, etc.   [ ]
c. Can wash self if prompted and supervised   [ ]
d. Unable to wash self and needs full assistance   [ ]
e. Not applicable   [ ]

7. Teeth
a. Cleans own teeth/dentures regularly and independently   [ ]
b. Cleans teeth/dentures if given appropriate items   [ ]
c. Requires some assistance, toothpaste on brush, brush to mouth, etc.   [ ]
d. Full assistance given   [ ]
e. Not applicable   [ ]

8. Bath/shower
a. Bathes regularly and independently   [ ]
b. Needs bath to be drawn/shower turned on but washes independently   [ ]
c. Needs supervision and prompting to wash   [ ]
d. Totally dependent, needs full assistance   [ ]
e. Not applicable   [ ]

9. Toilet/commode
a. Uses toilet appropriately when required   [ ]
b. Needs to be taken to the toilet and given assistance   [ ]
c. Incontinent of urine or faeces
d. Incontinent of urine and faeces   [ ]
e. Not applicable   [ ]

10. Transfers
a. Can get in/out of chair unaided   [ ]
b. Can get into a chair but needs help to get out   [ ]
c. Needs help getting in and out of a chair   [ ]
d. Totally dependent on being put into and lifted from chair   [ ]
e. Not applicable   [ ]

11. Mobility
a. Walks independently   [ ]
b. Walks with assistance, i.e. furniture, arm for support   [ ]
c. Uses aids to mobilize, i.e. frame, sticks etc.   [ ]
d. Unable to walk   [ ]
e. Not applicable   [ ]

12. Orientation – time
a. Fully orientated to time/day/date etc.   [ ]

b. *Unaware of time/day etc. but seems
    unconcerned*   [ ]
c. *Repeatedly asks the time/day/date*   [ ]
d. *Mixes up night and day*   [ ]
e. *Not applicable*   [ ]
13. Orientation – space
a. *Fully orientated to surroundings*   [ ]
b. *Orientated to familiar surroundings only*   [ ]
c. *Gets lost in home, needs reminding
    where bathroom is, etc.*   [ ]
d. *Does not recognize home as own and
    attempts to leave*   [ ]
e. *Not applicable*   [ ]

14. Communication
a. *Able to hold appropriate conversation*   [ ]
b. *Shows understanding and attempts to
    respond verbally with gestures*   [ ]
c. *Can make self understood but difficulty
    understanding others*   [ ]
d. *Does not respond to or communicate
    with others*   [ ]
e. *Not applicable*   [ ]

15. Telephone
a. *Uses telephone appropriately, including
    obtaining correct number*   [ ]
b. *Uses telephone if number given verbally
    /visually or predialled*   [ ]
c. *Answers telephone but does not make
    calls*   [ ]
d. *Unable/unwilling to use telephone at all*   [ ]
e. *Not applicable*   [ ]

16. Housework/gardening
a. *Able to do housework/gardening to
    previous standard*   [ ]
b. *Able to do housework/gardening but
    not to previous standard*   [ ]
c. *Limited participation even with a lot of
    supervision*   [ ]
d. *Unwilling/unable to participate in
    previous activities*   [ ]

e. *Not applicable*   [ ]
17. Shopping
a. *Shops to previous standard*   [ ]
b. *Only able to shop for 1 or 2 items with
    or without a list*   [ ]
c. *Unable to shop alone, but participates
    when accompanied*   [ ]
d. *Unable to participate in shopping even when
    accompanied*   [ ]
e. *Not applicable*   [ ]

18. Finances
a. *Responsible for own finances at
    previous level*   [ ]
b. *Unable to write cheque but can sign
    name and recognizes money values*   [ ]
c. *Can sign name but unable to recognize money
    values*   [ ]
d. *Unable to sign name or recognize
    money values*   [ ]
e. *Not applicable*   [ ]

19. Games/hobbies
a. *Participates in pastimes/activities to
    previous standard*   [ ]
b. *Participates but needs instruction/
    supervision*   [ ]
c. *Reluctant to join in, very slow, needs coaxing*   [ ]
d. *No longer able or willing to join in*   [ ]
e. *Not applicable*   [ ]

20. Transport
a. *Able to drive, cycle or use public
    transport independently*   [ ]
b. *Unable to drive but uses public
    transport or bike etc.*   [ ]
c. *Unable to use public transport alone*   [ ]
d. *Unable or unwilling to use transport
    even when accompanied*   [ ]
e. *Not applicable*   [ ]

Rating:
Tick only 1 box per activity. Answer with respect to last 2 weeks
Score: a 5 0, b 5 1, c 5 2, d 5 3, e 5 0

Reprinted from Bucks RS, Ashworth DL, Wilcock GK, Siegfried K (1996) Assessment of activities of daily living in dementia: development of the Bristol Activities of Daily Living Scale. *Age and Ageing,* 25: 113–20. By kind permission of Oxford University Press.

Geriatric Depression Scale (GDS)

Choose the best answer for how you felt the past week

1. Are you basically satisfied with your life?
2. Have you dropped many of your activities and interests?
3. Do you feel that your life is empty?
4. Do you often get bored?
5. Are you hopeful about the future?
6. Are you bothered by thoughts you can't get out of your head?
7. Are you in good spirits most of the time?
8. Are you afraid that something bad is going to happen to you?
9. Do you feel happy most of the time?
10. Do you often feel helpless?
11. Do you often get restless and fidgety?
12. Do you prefer to stay at home, rather than going out and doing new things?
13. Do you frequently worry about the future?
14. Do you feel you have more problems with memory than most?
15. Do you think it is wonderful to be alive now?
16. Do you often feel downhearted and blue?
17. Do you feel pretty worthless the way you are now?
18. Do you worry a lot about the past?
19. Do you find life very exciting?
20. Is it hard for you to get started on new projects?
21. Do you feel full of energy?
22. Do you feel that your situation is hopeless?
23. Do you think that most people are better off than you are?
24. Do you frequently get upset over little things?
25. Do you frequently feel like crying?
26. Do you have trouble concentrating?
27. Do you enjoy getting up in the morning?
28. Do you prefer to avoid social gatherings?
29. Is it easy for you to make decisions?
30. Is your mind as clear as it used to be?

Code answers as Yes or No

Score 1 for Yes on: 2–4,6,8,10–14,16–18,20,22–26,28
Score 1 for No on: 1,5,7,9,15,19,21,27,29,30

0–10 = Not depressed
11–20 = Mild depression
21–30 = Severe depression
GDS 15: 1,2,3,4,7,8,9,10,12,14,15,17,21,22,23 *(cut-off of 5/6 indicates depression)*
GDS 10: 1,2,3,8,9,10,14,21,22,23
GDS 4: 1,3,8,9 *(cut-off of 1/2 indicates depression)*

Reprinted from *Journal of Psychiatric Research*, Vol. 17, Yesavage JA, Brink TL, Rose TL, Lum O, Huang V, Adey M, Leirer O, Development and validation of a geriatric depression scale: a preliminary report, 1983, with permission from Elsevier Science.

Functional Assessment Staging (FAST)

Yes	Months¹	No.	
——	————	——	1. *No difficulties, either subjectively or objectively.*
——	————	——	2. *Complains of forgetting location of objects; subjective work difficulties.*
——	————	——	3. *Decrease job functioning evident to coworkers; difficulty in traveling to new locations.*
——	————	——	4. *Decreased ability to perform complex tasks (e.g., planning dinner for guests; handling finances; marketing)*
——	————	——	5. *Requires assistance in choosing proper clothing.*
——	————	——	6a. *Difficulty putting clothing on properly.*
——	————	——	6b. *Unable to bathe properly; may develop fear of bathing.*
——	————	——	6c. *Inability to handle mechanics of toileting (i.e., forgets to flush, doesn't wipe properly).*
——	————	——	6d. *Urinary incontinence.*
——	————	——	6e. *Fecal incontinence.*
——	————	——	7a. *Ability to speak limited (1 to 5 words a day).*
——	————	——	7b. *All intelligible vocabulary lost.*
——	————	——	7c. *Nonambulatory.*
——	————	——	7d. *Unable to sit up independently.*
——	————	——	7e. *Unable to smile.*
——	————	——	7f. *Unable to hold head up.*

TESTER: _____   *COMMENTS:* _____

Note: Functional staging score = Highest ordinal value. ¹Number of months FAST stage deficit has been noted.

Reproduced from Reisberg B (1988) Functional assessment staging (FAST). *Psychopharmacology Bulletin* 24: 653–9. © by Barry Reisberg, MD.

Clinical Dementia Rating (CDR)

	None 0	Questionable 0.5	Impairment Mild 1	Moderate 2	Severe 3
Memory	No memory loss or slight inconstant forgetfulness	Consistent slight forgetfulness; partial recollection of events; "benign" forgetfulness	Moderate memory loss; more marked for recent events; defect interferes with everyday activities	Severe memory loss; only highly learned material retained; new material rapidly lost	Severe memory loss; only fragments remain
Orientation	Fully oriented	Fully oriented except for slight difficulty with time relationships	Moderate difficulty with time relationships; oriented for place at examination; may have geographic disorientation elsewhere	Severe difficulty with time relationships; usually disoriented to time, often to place	Oriented to person only
Judgment and Problem Solving	Solves everyday problems and handles business and financial affairs well; judgment good in relation to past performance	Slight impairment in solving problems, similarities, and differences	Moderate difficulty in handling problems, similarities, and differences; social judgment usually maintained	Severely impaired in handling problems, similarities, and differences; social judgment usually impaired	Unable to make judgments or solve problems
Community Affairs	Independent function at usual level in job, shopping, and volunteer and social groups	Slight impairment in these activities	Unable to function independently at these activities although may still be engaged in some; appears normal to casual inspection	No pretense of independent function outside home Appears well enough to be taken to functions outside a family home	Appears too ill to be taken to functions outside a family home
Home and Hobbies	Life at home, hobbies, and intellectual interests well maintained	Life at home, hobbies, and intellectual interests slightly impaired	Mild but definite impairment of function at home; more difficult chores abandoned; more complicated hobbies and interests abandoned	Only simple chores preserved; very restricted interests, poorly maintained	No significant function in home
Personal Care	Fully capable of self-care		Needs prompting	Requires assistance in dressing, hygiene, keeping of personal effects	Requires much help with personal care; frequent incontinence

Rating:
Score only as decline from previous usual level due to cognitive loss, not impairment due to other factors

Reproduced from the *British Journal of Psychiatry*, Huges CP, Berg L, Danziger WL, Coben LA, Martin RL (1982) A new clinical scale for the staging of dementia. Vol. 140, pp. 566–72. © 1982 Royal College of Psychiatrists. Reproduced with permission.

Burden Interview

Reference   Zarit SH, Reever KE, Bach-Petersen J (1980) Relatives of the impaired elderly: correlates of
feeling of burden. *The Gerontologist* **20**: 649–55

Time taken   25 minutes (reviewer's estimate)
Rating   by self-report during an assessment
interview

Main indications
Assessment of the feelings of burden of caregivers in
caring for an older person with dementia.

Commentary
Twenty-nine patients with senile dementia and their
caregivers were interviewed, and the Burden
Interview was compared with measures of cognitive
function (Khan Mental Status Questionnaire; Khan
et al, 1960), a measure of mental state (Jacobs et al,
1977), a measure of the Memory and Problems
Checklist and activities of daily living as assessed by
scales described by Lawton (1971). The amount of
burden assessed was found to be less when more
visits were made by carers to the patient with
dementia, and severity of behavioural problems was
not associated with higher levels of burden. The
paper was one of the earlier studies to underscore
the importance of providing support to caregivers in
the community care of older people with dementia.

Additional references
Jacobs JW, Bernhard JR, Delgado A et al (1977)
Screening for organic mental syndromes in the
medically ill. *Annals of Internal Medicine* **86**: 40–6.

Khan RL, Goldfarb AI, Pollack J et al (1960) A
brief objective measure for the determination of
mental status of the aged. *American Journal of
Psychiatry* **117**: 326–8.

Lawton MP (1971) The functional assessment of
elderly people. *Journal of the American Geriatrics
Society* **19**: 465–80.

Address for correspondence
Steve Zarit
Gerontology Center
College of Health and Human Development
Pennsylvania State University
105 Henderson Building South
University Park
PA 16802–6500
USA

Burden Interview

1. I feel resentful of other relatives who could but who do not do things for my spouse.
2. I feel that my spouse makes requests which I perceive to be over and above what s/he needs.
3. Because of my involvement with my spouse, I don't have enough time for myself.
4. I feel stressed between trying to give to my spouse as well as to other family responsibilities, job, etc.
5. I feel embarrassed over my spouse's behavior.
6. I feel guilty about my interactions with my spouse.
7. I feel that I don't do as much for my spouse as I could or should.
8. I feel angry about my interactions with my spouse.
9. I feel that in the past, I haven't done as much for my spouse as I could have or should have.
10. I feel nervous or depressed about my interactions with my spouse.
11. I feel that my spouse currently affects my relationships with other family members and friends in a negative way.
12. I feel resentful about my interactions with my spouse.
13. I am afraid of what the future holds for my spouse.
14. I feel pleased about my interactions with my spouse.
15. It's painful to watch my spouse age.
16. I feel useful in my interactions with my spouse.
17. I feel my spouse is dependent.
18. I feel strained in my interactions with my spouse.
19. I feel that my health has suffered because of my involvement with my spouse.
20. I feel that I am contributing to the well-being of my spouse.
21. I feel that the present situation with my spouse doesn't allow me as much privacy as I'd like.
22. I feel that my social life has suffered because of my involvement with my spouse.
23. I wish that my spouse and I had a better relationship.
24. I feel that my spouse doesn't appreciate what I do for him/her as much as I would like.
25. I feel uncomfortable when I have friends over.
26. I feel that my spouse tries to manipulate me.
27. I feel that my spouse seems to expect me to take care of him/her as if I were the only one he/she could depend on.
28. I feel that I don't have enough money to support my spouse in addition to the rest of our expenses.
29. I feel that I would like to be able to provide more money to support my spouse than I am able to now.

ADCS–CLINICAL GLOBAL IMPRESSION OF CHANGE WORKSHEETS
Part 1–BASELINE CGIC Evaluation for both Subject and Informant

SUBJECT MUST BE INTERVIEWED FIRST

Subject Initials: _____ Subject ID: IN- __-__ Examiner Initials: _____ Date: _____

Time of day interview started: _____ (24 hour clock)

Brief Instructions: See instruction sheet. Use this form to record baseline information for assessing change at a later date. Information can be obtained from all relevant sources, including subject, informant, and staff members. A brief clinical assessment of mental state should be made. No particular format or order is suggested for the interview.

Area	Probes	Notes
Relevant history	recent relevant clinical events, illnesses?	Subject
		Informant
Observation/ Evaluation	appearance	Subject
		Informant

MENTAL/COGNITIVE STATE (Structured exam, if used: _____)

Arousal/ Alertness/ Attention/ Concentration	confusion/clarity excitement/reactivity state of consciousness	Subject
		Informant

Clinician's Global Impression of Change (CGIC)
Alzheimer's Disease Cooperative Study
A Multicenter Evaluation of New Treatment Efficacy Instruments for AD
Clinical Trials
Clinical Global Impression of Change – Summary Sheet
Baseline Visit

Center Name	Subject Number	Subject Initials	Examiner Initials	Examination Date
	IN-☐☐☐	☐☐☐	☐☐☐	☐☐ ☐☐ ☐☐☐☐ Month Day Year

1. Order of Administration
   ☐ Subject first, Informant second
   ☐ Informant first, Subject second

2. Time of day interview started:
   ☐☐ ☐☐ (24 hour clock)

3. The following sources of information were used in completing this assessment (check all that apply)
   ☐ Interview/examination of subject
   ☐ Interview of Informant
   ☐ Information on neuropsychological test performance
   ☐ General information derived from a staff conference about subject
   ☐ Other, please specify: _____

Area	Probes	Notes	
Orientation	time place person	Subject	
		Informant	
Memory	registration recall long term/remote recall for past events	Subject	
		Informant	
Language/ Speech	fluency/ expressive language receptive language comprehension paraphasia/word finding naming, amount repetition follows directions	Subject	
		Informant	
Praxis	constructional ability ideational praxis ideomotor/imitation	Subject	
		Informant	

Area	Probes	Notes	
Judgment/ Problem solving/ Insight	patient's behaviour in situations requiring judgment	Subject	
		Informant	
BEHAVIOUR			
Thought content	organization appropriateness	Subject	
		Informant	
Hallucinations/ Delusions/ Illusions	auditory/visual misperceptions systematized/developed	Subject	
		Informant	
Behaviour/Mood	affect/lability unusual/bizarre uninhibited motivation/energy wandering/getting lost agitation/aggression hostility depression-related anxiety-related appropriateness cooperativeness	Subject	
		Informant	

Area	Probes	Notes	
Sleep/Appetite	sleep disorder insomnia (type?) nocturnal activity hyper-, hyposomnia appetite/weight change	Subject	
		Informant	
Neurological/ Psychomotor activity	overall motor activity postural/gait movement disorder unusual motor behaviour daily patterns	Subject	
		Informant	
FUNCTIONING			
Basic and complex Instrumental/ functional ability	mobility hygiene/grooming dressing self-feeding shopping household chores/hobbies finances driving	Subject	
		Informant	
Social function	participation in: social interactions community activities independence helplessness	Subject	
		Informant	

Notes, comments, summary statement:

Information from other sources:

The following sources of information were used in completing this form:

— Interview/examination of subject

— Interview of informant. Describe relationship to subject: _____

— Information on neuropsychological test performance

— General information derived from a staff conference about the subject

— Other: _____

DISABILITY ASSESSMENT FOR DEMENTIA (DAD)

Authors: L Gauthier and I Gélinas
Collaborators: M McIntyre, S Gauthier,
                    H Laberge and S Wood
                    Dauphinee

Introduction

The literature as well as consultations with health care professionals and caregivers clearly indicates the need for a disability measure designed specifically for community-dwelling individuals with dementia of the Alzheimer type (DAT). Such an instrument is essential to help clinicians and caregivers make decisions regarding the choice of suitable interventions and to monitor disease progression. In addition, as a research tool, it could be used to describe the functional characteristics of populations with DAT, the course of the disease and also as an outcome variable in intervention studies and clinical trials. The Disability Assessment for Dementia (DAD) Scale was developed in an attempt to fulfill these needs.

Objectives of the DAD

The objectives of the DAD Scale are to quantitatively measure functional abilities in activities of daily living (ADL) in individuals with cognitive impairments such as dementia and to help delineate areas of cognitive deficits which may impair performance in ADL. Basic and instrumental activities of daily living are examined in relation to executive skills to permit identification of the problematic areas. The primary aim is to have a standardized, valid, reliable and sensitive measure of functional disability in DAT and other dementias. Another objective is to obtain a French and English instrument which is short and easy to administer.

Target population

The DAD Scale is intended specifically for the assessment of disability in community residing individuals with cognitive deficits such as DAT and other dementias. This tool has not been designed to meet the specific needs of populations with physical disabilities (neuro-muscular deficits). In cases where an individual will present both cognitive and physical deficits which may impair function in ADL, this tool should not be used exclusively but rather in conjunction with another assessment of ADL designed for physical disabilities.

DISABILITY ASSESSMENT FOR DEMENTIA (DAD)

Name:			File No:	
Date:	MMS:	GDS:	DAD:	
Respondent:		Relationship:		
Specify all motor and sensory disorders:				
Rater:			Time:	

During the past two weeks, did (name) _____, without help or reminder *HYGIENE* SCORING: YES = 1 NO = 0 N/A = Not Applicable	Initiation	Planning & Organization	Effective Performance
Undertake to wash himself/herself or to take a bath or a shower			
Undertake to brush his/her teeth or care for his/her dentures			
Decide to care for his/her hair (wash and comb)			
Prepare the water, towels, and soap for washing, taking a bath or a shower			
Wash and dry completely all parts of his/her body safely			
Brush his/her teeth or care for his/her dentures appropriately			
Care for his/her hair (wash and comb)			
DRESSING			
Undertake to dress himself/herself			
Choose appropriate clothing (with regard to the occasion, neatness, the weather and color combination)			
Dress himself/herself in the appropriate order (undergarments, pant/dress, shoes)			
Dress himself/herself completely			
Undress himself/herself completely			
CONTINENCE			
Decide to use the toilet at appropriate times			
Use the toilet without "accidents"			
EATING			
Decide that he/she needs to eat			
Choose appropriate utensils and seasonings when eating			
Eat his/her meals at a normal pace and with appropriate manners			
MEAL PREPARATION			
Undertake to prepare a light meal or snack for himself/herself			
Adequately plan a light meal or snack (ingredients, cookware)			
Prepare or cook a light meal or a snack safely			
TELEPHONING			
Attempt to telephone someone at a suitable time			
Find and dial a telephone number correctly			
Carry out an appropriate telephone conversation			
Write and convey a telephone message adequately			

During the past two weeks, did (name) _____, without help or reminder

	Initiation	Planning & Organization	Effective Performance

GOING ON AN OUTING   SCORING: YES=1   NO=0   N/A=Not Applicable

Undertake to go out (walk, visit, shop) at an appropriate time

Adequately organize an outing with respect to transportation, keys, destination, weather, necessary money, shopping list

Go out and reach a familiar destination without getting lost

Safely take the adequate mode of transportation (car, bus, taxi)

Return from the store with the appropriate items

FINANCE AND CORRESPONDENCE

Show an interest in his/her finances and written correspondence

Organize his/her finance to pay his/her bills (cheques, bankbook, bills)

Adequately organize his/her correspondence with respect to stationery, address, stamps

Handle adequately his/her money (make change)

MEDICATIONS

Decide to take his/her medications at the correct time

Take his/her medications as prescribed (according to the right dosage)

LEISURE AND HOUSEWORK

Show an interest in leisure activity(ies)

Take an interest in household chores that he/she used to perform in the past

Plan and organize adequately household chores that he/she used to perform in the past

Complete household chores adequately as he/she used to perform in the past

Stay safely at home by himself/herself when needed

Comments:

	Initiation	Planning & Organization	Effective Performance
SUB TOTAL/#applicable items	/	/	/
DAD TOTAL/#applicable items	/		
DAD TOTAL in %			

References

Alexopoulos GS, Abrams RC, Young RC, Shamoian CA (1988). Cornell scale for depression in dementia. *Biol Psychiatry* 23, 271–84.

Ballard C, Fossey J, Chithramohan R, , et al (2001). Quality of care in private sector and NHS facilities for people with dementia: cross sectional survey. *BMJ* 323, 426–7.

Bedard M, Molloy DW, Squire L, Dubois S, Lever JA, O'Donnell M (2001). The Zarit Burden Interview: a new short version and screening version. *Gerontologist*. 41, 652–7.

Bowie P, Branton T, Holmes J (1999). Should the Mini Mental State Examination be used to monitor dementia treatment? *Lancet* 354, 1527–8.

Brodaty H, Moore CM (1997). The Clock Drawing Test for dementia of the Alzheimer type: a comparison of 3 scoring methods in a memory disorders clinic. *Int J Geriat Psychiatry* 12, 619–27.

Brooker D (2005). Dementia care mapping: a review of the research literature. *Gerontologist* 4, 11–8.

Bucks RS, Ashworth DL, Wilcock GK, Siegfried K (1996). Assessment of activities of daily living in dementia: development of the Bristol Activities of Daily Living Scale. *Age Ageing* 25, 113–20.

Burns A, Lawlor B, Craig S (2004). *Assessment scales on old age psychiatry*, 2nd edn. London, UK: Martin Dunitz.

Cohen-Mansfield J, Marx MS, Rosenthal AS (1989). A description of agitation in a nursing home. *J Gerontol Med Sci* 4, M77–84.

Devanand DP, Miller L, Richards M, et al (1992). The Columbia University Scale for Psychopathology in Alzheimer's disease. *Arch Neurol*. 49, 371–6.

Fillenbaum GG, Peterson B, Morris JC (1996). Estimating the validity of the clinical Dementia Rating Scale: the CERAD experience. Consortium to Establish a Registry for Alzheimer's Disease. *Aging Clin Exp Res* 8, 379–85.

Folstein MF, Folstein SE, McHugh PR (1975). 'Mini-mental state.' A practical method for grading the cognitive state of patients for the clinician. *J Psychiatr Res* 12, 189–98.

Fossey J, Lee L, Ballard C (2002). Dementia Care Mapping as a research tool for measuring quality of life in care settings: psychometric properties. *Int J Geriat Psychiatry*. 17, 1064–70.

Galasko D, Bennett D, Sano M, et al (1997). An inventory to assess activities of daily living for clinical trials in Alzheimer's disease. The Alzheimer's Disease Cooperative Study. *Alzheimer Dis Assoc Disord* 11(suppl 2), S33–9.

Gélinas I, Gauthier L, McIntyre M, Gauthier S (1999). Development of a functional measure for persons with Alzheimer's disease: the disability assessment for dementia. *Am J Occup Ther* 53, 471–81.

Hope T, Fairburn CG (1992). The Present Behavioural Examination (PBE): the development of an interview to measure current behaviour abnormalities. *Psychol Med* 22, 223–30.

Kitwood T, Bredin K (1997). *Evaluating dementia care the DCM method*, 7th edn. Bradford, UK: Bradford Dementia Research Group, Bradford University.

Logsdon RG, Gibbons LE, McCurry SM, Teri L (2002). Assessing quality of life in older adults with cognitive impairment. *Psychosom Med*. 64, 510–9.

Nasreddine ZS, Phillips NA, Bedirian V, et al (2005). The Montreal Cognitive Assessment, MoCA: a brief screening tool for mild cognitive impairment. *J Am Geriatr Soc* 53, 695–9.

Patel V, Hope RA (1992). A rating scale for aggressive behaviour in the elderly – the RAGE. *Psychol Med* 22, 211–21.

Reisberg B (1988). Functional assessment staging (FAST). *Psychopharmacol Bull* 24, 653–9.

Reynolds T, Thornicroft G, Abas M, et al (2000). Camberwell Assessment of Need for the Elderly (CANE). Development, validity and reliability. *Br J Psychiatry* 176, 444–52.

Rosen WG, Mohs RC, Davis KL (1984). A new rating scale for Alzheimer's disease. *Am J Psychiatry* 141, 1356–64.

Royall DR, Cordes JA, Polk M (1998). CLOX: an executive clock drawing task. *J Neurol Neurosurg Psychiatry* 64, 588–94.

Royall DR, Mahurin RK, Gray K (1992). Bedside assessment of executive cognitive impairment: the executive interview (EXIT). *J Am Geriatr Soc* 40, 1221–6.

Saxton J, McGonigle-Gibson K, Swihart A, Miller M, Boller F (1990). Assessment of severely impaired patients: description and validation of a new neuropsychological test battery. *Psychol Assess* 2, 298–303.

Schneider LS, Olin JT, Doody RS, et al (1997). Validity and reliability of the Alzheimer's Disease Cooperative Study-Clinical Global Impression of Change. The Alzheimer's Disease Cooperative Study. *Alzheimer Dis Assoc Disord* 11(suppl 2), S22–32.

Shankar KK, Walker M, Frost D, Orrell MW (1999) The development of a reliable and valid scale for rating anxiety in dementia (RAID). *Aging Ment Health* 3, 39–49.

Smith SC, Lamping DL, Banerjee S, et al (2007). Development of a new measure of health-related quality of life for people with dementia: DEMQOL. *Psychol Med* 37, 737–46.

Starkstein SE, Migliorelli R, Manes F, et al (1995). The prevalence and clinical correlates of apathy and irritability in Alzheimer's disease. *Eur J Neurol* 2, 540–6.

Future perspectives

10

This book is aimed at outlining the components of a comprehensive management of Alzheimer's disease (AD) through its different stages, with additional discussion about other dementias where appropriate. Both non-pharmacological and pharmacological approaches have been considered, with the best evidence available at this time (Table 10.1).

What we hope to see in the near future is earlier diagnosis using validated diagnostic criteria for 'pre-dementia' AD (Dubois et al, 2007) and successful disease-modifying strategies that may well be different at asymptomatic, early symptomatic and different stages of dementia (Cummings et al, 2007). Furthermore there may be phenotypic (age of onset of symptoms, patterns of early symptoms, associated clinical features) and genotypic characteristics that will guide selection among diverse disease-modifying therapies for each individual. To make this possible, 'responder analysis' is very much part of all ongoing clinical trials, whether primarily aiming for symptomatic or disease-modifying effects. In other words, it may well be that a class of drugs such as statins may exert a disease-modifying effect if taken before dementia is

Table 10.1
*Current management of AD across stages**

Stage of AD	GDS**	Clinical management
Asymptomatic 'at risk'	1	Control of risk factors
Subjective cognitive complaints	2	+ look for depression, anxiety
MCI/'pre-dementia'AD	3	+ monitor closely for functional decline
Mild dementia	4	Standard symptomatic treatment (CIs)
Moderate dementia	5	+ memantine; monitor for emerging BPSD
Severe dementia	6	+ BPSD therapies
Terminal stage	7	Palliative care, pain relief

*Modified from Gauthier & Poirier, 2008.
**Global Deterioration Scale, Reisberg et al, 1982.
Abbreviations: CIs, cholinesterase inhibitors; BPSD, behavioral and psychological symptoms in dementia.

clinically manifested and be effective only in a subgroup of subjects based on ApoE genotype. This pharmacogenomic approach (Poirier & Gauthier, 2008) may well be the key to clinical acceptance of a long treatment prior to dementia, and to reimbursement by third-party payers. Another possible finding is that the age matters in terms of treatment; the amyloid load is more likely to be a key factor in young persons with AD (< 65 years) than older ones (> 75 years) where cerebrovascular and Lewy body co-morbidity is prominent. Hence amyloid-targeted therapies may be most useful in early onset AD. We will know within the next two years, as many randomised clinical trials are underway in the traditional 'dementia of AD type'. We predict that successful trials at that stage of AD will be quickly followed by trials in pre-dementia

stages, where there is more likely a chance at brain recovery. It will also be important to focus similar clinical trials and specific targeted therapies at the secondary prevention of dementia in other groups of individuals at substantially increased risk of progressive cognitive decline, such as patients experiencing a stroke.

In terms of primary prevention, there is interest in establishing a 'risk score' as early as 'midlife' (Kivipelto et al, 2006), in a way similar to establishing the risk of cardiovascular disease. Hopefully, there will be sufficient evidence from prospective studies to provide useful advice about lifestyle changes that will reduce the risk of AD, with or without diet and antioxidant supplementation (Panel 10.1).

Some international multi-sites studies are under planning to establish if individual or

Panel 10.1

Potential lifestyle changes, diet/antioxidant supplementation and treatment of medical problems that may decrease the risk of AD and other dementias in persons at risk*

> - *physical exercise*
> - *weight reduction*
> - *control of hypertension*
> - *control of hypercholesterolaemia*
> - *dietary antioxidants*
> - *intellectual activity*
> - *leisure activities & hobbies*
> - *social networks*
> - *red wine*
> - *fish and other sources of ω3*
> - *folate-rich food or low-dose supplementation*
>
> ---
>
> **All these need to be validated prospectively and should be used in moderation.*

combination of life-style changes reduce the risk of cognitive decline with age and incident dementia (Vellas et al, 2008).

What until then? There has been much progress in the management of dementia, and interested health professionals have seen benefit of this management over the past decade. There is cause for optimism in the treatment of AD and related disorders.

References

Cummings JL, Doody R, Clark C (2007). Disease-modifying therapies for Alzheimer's disease. *Neurology* 69, 1622–34.

Dubois B, Feldman HH, Jacova C, et al (2007). Research criteria for the diagnosis of Alzheimer's disease: revising the NINCDS-ADRDA criteria. *Lancet Neurol* 6, 734–46.

Gauthier S, Poirier J (2008). Current and future management of Alzheimer's disease. *Alzheimers Dement* 4, S48–50.

Kivipelto M, Ngandu T, Laatikainen T, Winblad B, Soininen H, Tuomilehto J (2006). Risk score for the prediction of dementia risk in 20 years among middle aged people: a longitudinal, population-based study. *Lancet Neurol* 5, 735–41.

Poirier J, Gauthier S (2008). Pharmacogenomics and the treatment of sporadic Alzheimer's disease: a decade of progress. *Curr Pharmacogenom Personal Med* 6, 63–76.

Reisberg B, Ferris SH, de Leon MJ, Crook T (1982). The Global Deterioration Scale (GDS) for assessment of primary degenerative dementia. *Am J Psychiatry* 139, 1136–9.

Vellas B, Gillette-Guyonnet S, Andrieu S (2008). Memory health-clinics – a first step to prevention. *Alzheimers Dement* 4, S144–9.

Appendix

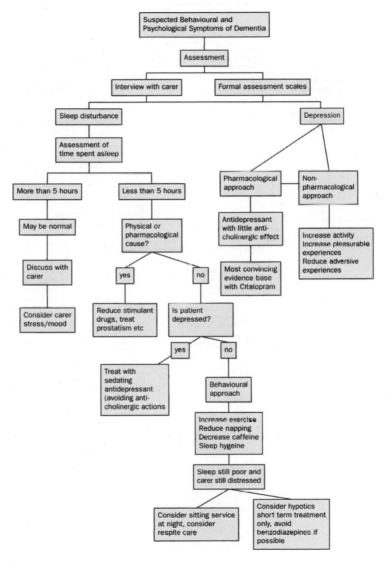

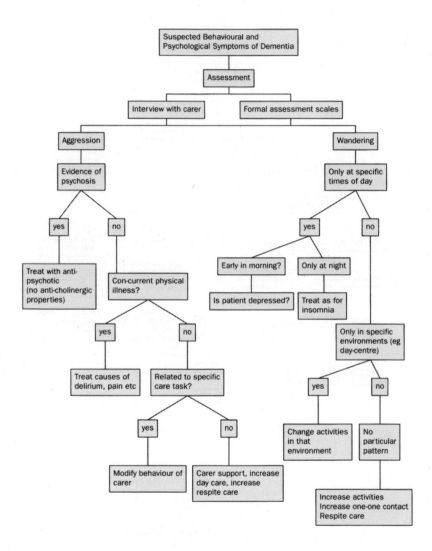

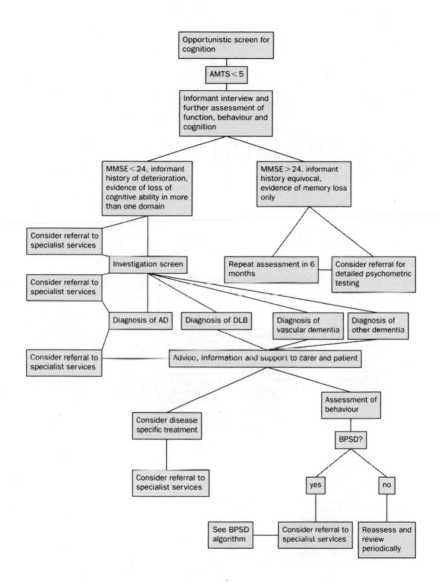

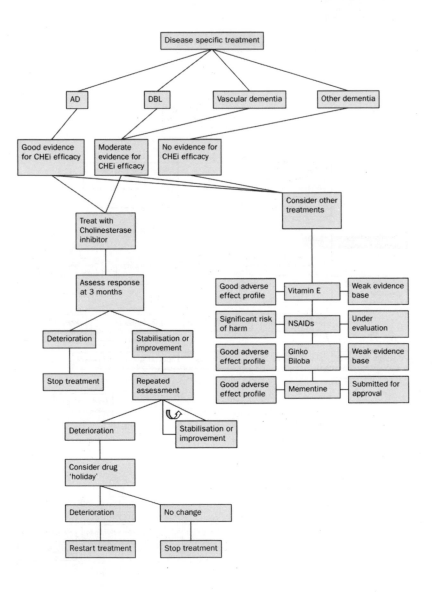

Index